MORE THAN JUST A
PRETTY FACE
LIVING IN BEAUTIFUL OBEDIENCE

MORE THAN JUST A
PRETTY FACE
LIVING IN BEAUTIFUL OBEDIENCE

KAREN MOREROD

Advancing the Ministries of the Gospel

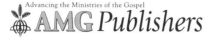 AMG *Publishers*

God's Word to you is our highest calling.

More Than Just a Pretty Face: The Beauty of Obedience

© 2011 by Karen Morerod

Published by AMG Bible Studies. All Rights Reserved.

First Printing, September 2011

Print Edition	ISBN 13: 978-0-89957-017-4	ISBN 10: 0-89957-017-8
EPUB Edition	ISBN 13: 978-1-61715-304-4	ISBN 10: 1-61715-304-4
Mobi Edition	ISBN 13: 978-1-61715-305-1	ISBN 10: 1-61715-305-2
E-PDF Edition	ISBN 13: 978-1-61715-306-8	ISBN 10: 1-61715-306-0

Edited by Diane Stortz and Rick Steele

Layout by Adept Content Solutions, Urbana, Illinois

Front cover design by Taylor Ware, InView Graphics, Chattanooga, Tennessee

Cover layout by Michael Largent, InView Graphics, Chattanooga, Tennessee

Printed in the United States of America

16 15 14 13 12 11 –R– 6 5 4 3 2 1

CONTENTS

INTRODUCTION

BEAUTY ANALYSIS

I sat on the bleachers at the ballpark and watched my Little Leaguer. Another mother sat nearby, and I suspiciously eyed her golden, bronzed appendages and wondered, *Is that tan real?*

I chided my critical attitude and tried to refocus on the game, until I noticed another mom. Her silky hair fluttered as she bounded like a gazelle to her place three rows above me. How did she get her hair like that? I tucked my wavy, coarse hair behind my ears.

Within moments, another woman pranced in with, as usual, a perfect outfit, coordinated with necklace and earrings.

Before you could say, "Mirror, mirror on the wall," my eyes darted around and analyzed every other female in the grandstands. Tanner. Skinnier. Silkier. Me? Pale. Frizzy. And poster child for Chocolate Overeaters Anonymous.

I reviewed my options at this point:

A. Have my son join another team.

B. Bring homemade cinnamon rolls to every game—maybe all the moms would gain twenty pounds.

C. Wear a shirt that said, "BODY NOT AS BIG AS IT APPEARS."

Momentary consideration rendered the verdict that God probably wouldn't look too highly on these options. Then I panicked. I thought, *I sure need another source of beauty because this outside beauty thing isn't going so well.*

Since that day, I have often had to remind myself: outward beauty does not guarantee happiness or contentment. I knew some of these women had challenging lives. But that seemed to be a smaller issue than what I knew deep down: God has higher concerns for me than my outward appearance.

Queen Esther's beauty won the king's heart and landed her a spot as First Lady of Persia. But when I read about her in the Bible, I asked myself whether her beauty had any part in her courage to go to the king to expose an evil plot. Did all those oil treatments give her wisdom for making critical decisions? Did Esther's good looks help her confront the arrogant Haman? Surely she must have had another source of strength to accomplish her task.

Then I pondered: Esther must have realized life is more than just manicures and dieting. She was most beautiful to God when she was obedient to him. Could a closer relationship to God cause me to radiate beauty equal to that of the lovely Queen Esther? What if my obedience to God was my beauty?

For the next thirty-one days, I hope you'll smile as we peek at our culture's crazy attempts at beauty—as well as some not-so-brilliant efforts by yours truly. Then as we study Queen Esther, we'll discover how to follow God more closely and become the genuinely beautiful women he created us to be.

Our cast includes the following characters:

King Xerxes, the prideful, powerful, yet willing-to-right-a-wrong king of Persia;

Queen Vashti, his wife, who refused to report and then reaped the results;

Haman, high official at the palace and schemer of all things deceitful and prideful;

Mordecai, award-winning cousin of the year and doer of all things good and right; and

Esther, orphan-turned-royalty star of the show.

We know Esther was beautiful and the King thought she was hot. But there must have been something deeper.

Was it Botox?

And Esther won the favor of everyone who saw her.

—Esther 2:15

MY FOUNDATION

PART 1

THE PLAN

APPLYING FOUNDATION

THE BOTTOM LINE

I gazed at the foundation selection in the cosmetic department. What was the color I bought last time? I scanned the choices: ivory, classic ivory, natural ivory, creamy natural, buff beige, classic beige, natural beige, warm beige, creamy beige. And that was just the first row. Only Sherwin-Williams could compete with all those colors.

I'd always been told that foundation choice is vital. Even the word itself sounds, um, well, foundational. So I did what any woman of my caliber of beauty expertise would do. I closed my eyes and said, "Eenie, meenie, miney, moe."

Several days later an Internet ad popped up that said, "Foundation Specialists." I clicked to research. The website read, "Are your walls cracking or bowing?"

Well, wrinkles—maybe. But cracks? Sounds a bit harsh.

Then I read, "Are your doors sticking?" and realized I must have taken a wrong turn in cyberspace. But you have to admit, "Foundation Specialists" sounds like something a girl could use occasionally.

Foundations are important—and not only the kind you buy in a bottle or the one that supports your home. God desires a relationship with us, and the foundation of that relationship needs to be Jesus Christ. As we build on that foundation, we can follow the plan he has for our lives.

The apostle Paul reminds us, **"Just as He chose us in Him before the foundation of the world, that we would be holy and blameless before Him. *In love He predestined us to adoption* as sons through Jesus Christ to Himself, according to the kind intention of His will** (Ephesians 1:4–5 NASB, emphasis mine).

There's that foundation thing again. Even before the foundation was set—the foundation of the world that God would create—God wanted a relationship with his people. And that is where all of our purposes intersect—a relationship with God through Jesus Christ.

Do you believe that God has a plan for your life? Do you wonder what that plan is? Or maybe you're wondering why God has your pretty face smack-dab in the middle of the life you're living right now.

Those can be tough questions, but we can know a couple things for sure.

First, God didn't go to all the trouble of creating the world and all humankind just for us to exist in misery. Oh, we're going to have problems within this plan called life, and we will touch more on this later. But God has a plan for us to live out. Consider these Scriptures:

"You saw me before I was born. Every day of my life was recorded in your book. Every moment was laid out before a single day had passed" (Psalm 139:16 NLT).

"For I know the plans I have for you," declares the Lord, "plans to prosper you and not to harm you, plans to give you hope and a future" (Jeremiah 29:11 NIV).

Second, we can know that God is indeed is offering us a foundation—a relationship with him. It's this foundation that allows us to live out the plan for which he created us.

THE ESTHER FACTOR

God certainly used Esther in a dramatic plan. But we have to wonder—the book of Esther never uses the word *God*, or *Jehovah*, the most common name in the Old Testament for *Lord*. We don't see Esther worshiping, talking about God, or even praying. However, she does fast when confronted with an overwhelming situation. And in biblical times, fasting by a Jew was consistent with prayer to Jehovah (God).

From the context and events, we can be confident Esther had a foundational relationship with her God. That is how she was able to carry out the plan God laid before her. She knew the source of her willingness and strength.

For any of us to live out God's plan, we first must have a relationship with the author of that plan. That's where it starts: acknowledging there is someone out there bigger than we are, and way more holy than we are, who will save us from our sinful selves and help us live out our intended purposes.

Is it easier for us to build a relationship with God than it was for Esther? We live two thousand years this side of Jesus Christ's coming to earth. We have historical and archeological evidence for the biblical account of God's Son. We have thousands of years of testimonies from people experiencing faith in Jesus. So if Esther could have faith in a God who had simply *promised* a redeemer, how much more can we believe with history on our side?

So how is your foundation? And not the kind in a bottle from the store. Is your life built on a relationship with God through Jesus Christ? If you've never laid that foundation for your life, see Applying the Foundation in the back of this book. It will show you the steps for beginning your life with God. It's one decision you will never regret. And much simpler than choosing the right foundation color.

> Later when the anger of King Xerxes had subsided, he
> remembered Vashti and what she had done and what

he had decreed about her. Then the king's personal
attendants proposed, "Let a search be made for
beautiful young virgins for the king. Let the king appoint
commissioners in every province of his realm to bring all
these beautiful girls into the harem at the citadel of Susa.
Let them be placed under the care of Hegai, the king's
eunuch, who is in charge of the women; and let beauty
treatments be given to them. Then let the girl who pleases
the king be queen instead of Vashti." This advice appealed
to the king, and he followed it.

—Esther 2:1–4 NIV

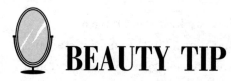 **BEAUTY TIP**

The foundation always goes on first.

MY FOUNDATION

MY FOUNDATION

What Lies Beneath

YOUR FOUNDATION'S MAKEUP

I met Cover Girl when I was ten years old.

"Hey, come over and play in the snow with us," hollered my neighbor Becky from her yard. I ran to get my sled, and we headed to the top of a hill between our yards.

I jumped on my round, aluminum sled. Becky gave me a twirl, and I spun down the hill. "Woo-hoo! This is fun!" I shrieked.

Suddenly, my spiraling fun turned into a smash finale on a fat tree trunk. Crying, I ran into the house to assess the damage to my face. "Oh no! I can't go to school like this," I moaned as I examined my swelling nose and the scrapes on my face.

But Mom had a secret. That next morning before school, she dabbed my multiple wounds with her faithful Cover Girl foundation, and I looked good as new. Or at least I thought no one would know what lay beneath my new, smooth facade. That was my first lesson in using makeup to cover a multitude of sins. Cover Girl worked wonders.

When we build a life foundation on Jesus Christ, it does much more than cover a multitude of sins. Of course I am extremely grateful that Jesus died to forgive all the wounds and sins of my life. But when we develop a deep relationship with Jesus Christ, we begin to see that we are each much more than a pretty face.

We weren't put here just to get saved and look cute!

After we lay the foundation and accept God's new life in Christ, we begin to see our value. How God created us. What we're wired to do. But many of us sabotage our own self-images. We become haunted by past mistakes and too intimidated to be all that God intends for us to be.

We think and say things like, "I'm not all that great. What do I have to offer?" Or, "I know God forgave me, but my past is so bad, I'll never be able to spiritually influence anyone else." Or the biggest lie, "I don't have any talents to really do anything for God."

With enemies like that, who needs Satan whispering in our ears?

The truth is that God has equipped each of us with exactly what we need to carry out whatever he intends. He is our makeup artist! Look at these different versions of Psalm 139:13:

"For you created my inmost being; you knit me together in my mother's womb" (NIV).

"You made all the delicate, inner parts of my body and knit me together in my mother's womb" (NLT).

"Oh yes, you first shaped me inside, then out; you formed me in my mother's womb" (MSG).

"You created the deepest parts of my being. You put me together inside my mother's body" (NIRV).

Oh yes, girlfriends, we need to know that how we're made and what we've experienced is for a reason. We might have experienced woundings, we might have emotional scars, and we might have once lived blatantly defiant lifestyles. Very likely we still have a few undesirable traits to work on. But God has this bizarre habit of creating something out of nothing and bringing good out of bad to accomplish his purposes!

One of the hardest prayers I've prayed is that I will see myself as God does. It's too bad I know myself so well. I recall every ugly thought, shameful action, and nasty word that's come out of my mouth. How could God love that?

But God sees the potential in me. He remembers the original plan for my life, how he wired me, and he is confident that, as I trust him, the one who sees beneath, I can do exactly what he purposed from the beginning.

THE ESTHER FACTOR

Esther had been brought to the palace as an addition to King Xerxes' harem as part of the search to find a replacement for Queen Vashti. It wasn't Cover Girl, but Esther experienced beauty treatments that would make any Miss America jealous: six months with oil of myrrh and six months with other perfumes and cosmetics, apparently at no cost to her.

This young maiden had no royal experience, no family wealth (she was an orphan), and definitely no degree from the Persia Institute of Beauty. Added to that, she was a different nationality from the king—a little secret her cousin Mordecai forbade her to disclose.

Did she ever think, *I'm just an orphan. I can't do this?* Or, *If they find out who I really am, they'll send me back faster than camel spit.* Or, *Really? Me? You've got to be kidding!* These thoughts aren't addressed in Scripture, but I believe Esther was a normal-thinking young girl. She likely had some insecurity.

But leave it to God. He took a most unlikely candidate and put a crown on her head. God saw beyond her past, above her insufficiencies, and through her outward beauty! Esther's position in time and place was no accident. And, by the way, neither is yours.

As the story progresses, we get a chance to see Esther's faith in action. There might have been days where she simply had to push through the task—scared but believing that Jehovah God really *was* in control.

God planned from the very beginning for Esther to be instrumental in the protection of his people. And he gifted her with whatever was necessary for her to carry out the mission.

> When the king's order and edict had been proclaimed, many girls were brought to the citadel of Susa and put under the care of Hegai. Esther also was taken to the king's palace and entrusted to Hegai, who had charge

of the harem. The girl pleased him and won his favor.
Immediately he provided her with her beauty treatments
and special food. He assigned to her seven maids selected
from the king's palace and moved her and her maids into
the best place in the harem.

Esther had not revealed her nationality and family
background, because Mordecai had forbidden her to do so.
Every day he walked back and forth near the courtyard
of the harem to find out how Esther was and what was
happening to her.

Before a girl's turn came to go in to King Xerxes,
she had to complete twelve months of beauty treatments
prescribed for the women, six months with oil of myrrh
and six with perfumes and cosmetics.

—Esther 2:8–12 (NIV84)

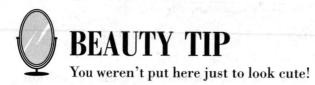

BEAUTY TIP

You weren't put here just to look cute!

MY FOUNDATION

MY FOUNDATION

IF YOU CAN'T GET AROUND IT, FACE IT

If only I could practice what I preach. I've often wondered what God thinks when we complain about the way he's made us. But I'm here to come clean to the fact that I have a complaint: I don't like the shape of my face. Is it more spiritually mature to say I question why God would want to give me such a round face? I mean, really, all I'm asking for is a slender, high-cheeked, triangular face.

Instead I have this round, pudgy mug. It's been confirmed several times over. One summer an artist friend drew caricatures at our church carnival, and of course I wanted a picture. However, it took everything within me not to break down and cry when he showed me the drawing. There I was, all chalked out on the poster—my round cheeks beaming all over the place, puffed out like a squirrel in nut-collecting season.

Sometime later I talked hairstyles with my good friend who is a cosmetologist. I had recently lost some weight, and, I told her, "I still don't like my face in photos. Isn't there a new hairstyle to complement my face?" Her words came down like a gavel in a courtroom: "We can change your hairstyle, but your face is always going to be round."

Alas.

OK, so I'm fifty. Maybe I should get over it because I can't get around it. It's time to face my face. God made it this way. I'm currently searching for a support group.

There's also a biblical truth we should face—God has a plan for us. And he has designed us the way we are physically, emotionally, spiritually, and mentally so we can live the life he intended. One of the many verses in the Bible that tells us this is **Ephesians 2:10: "For we** are God's workmanship, created in Christ Jesus to do good works, which God prepared in advance for us to do" (NIV84).

This is a loaded verse, but consider these two thoughts. First, the word *workmanship* suggests a work of art or a masterpiece. So, as we discussed in Day 2, God crafted us perfectly, inside and out. Evidently God is more concerned that I use the gifts and talents he gave than he is with the shape of my face. And that should be my priority—to function as his masterpiece, obeying his plan for my life.

Second, Ephesians 2:10 says God predetermined the things he wants me to do. He had my to-do list ready the day I took my first breath. I find this revolutionary! God has charted out my course, and I have a responsibility to seek him for this path. Even though there are bumps along the course, I'd rather experience difficulty within God's boundaries than wander aimlessly outside his loving plan for my life.

So I think I'll start by being thankful for the face I've been given and then continue to work on that to-do list, shining my little round face wherever I go!

The Esther Factor

Hmm . . . was Esther ever discontented with one of her physical features? There is no record of that, but I wonder if she ever questioned her to-do list.

The book of Esther doesn't give many concrete revelations about Esther's emotions or misgivings. However, we can observe two things. First, as Mordecai asks Esther to approach the king with a difficult request, we see her stern response. She reminds him of the danger of approaching the king without an invitation. She obviously had some serious questions about her safety. She probably even had doubts that this was actually her purpose in life. I can hear her saying, "God, this sounds extremely dangerous. Are you sure you want me to do this?"

Second, we see her admit she could die if she consents to visit the king at Mordecai's request. Yet she agrees to the mission, closing her letter with, "And if I perish, I perish." That's enough to worry the hair on any pretty little girl's head! But Esther carried out the task. She believed it was her calling and that she was indeed created to do it.

Not many of us will be faced with the threat of death because we follow God. So why do we cop out on many things that would bring honor and glory to God? We fail to tell a coworker we will pray for her during her difficulties. We don't engage in spiritual discussions with our neighbors or even invite them to church. And we neglect to share God's message of love, grace, and forgiveness, even with friends we know are not followers of Jesus.

What made Esther so willing, and why am I so hesitant? I don't know about you, but deep down I fear rejection or ridicule. Fearful that I won't be asked out to lunch at work. Anxious that other people will talk behind my back. Worried that a friend will think I'm a spiritual radical simply for inviting her to church. I bet Esther wished that rejection or ridicule was all she had at stake.

I don't think Esther had some magical secret that explains why she weighed her situation and then did what she was supposed to. She simply was a woman willing to face the plan God put before her and to be obedient no matter the cost. And that is probably one of the most outstanding truths from the book of Esther—what can be accomplished when a woman chooses to live a simple, beautifully obedient life.

> So Hathak went out to Mordecai in the open square of the city in front of the king's gate. Mordecai told him everything that had happened to him, including the exact amount of money Haman had promised to pay into the royal treasury for the destruction of the Jews. He also gave him a copy of the text of the edict for their annihilation, which had been published in Susa, to show to Esther and explain it to her, and he told him to instruct her to go into the king's presence to beg for mercy and plead with him for her people.
>
> Hathak went back and reported to Esther what Mordecai had said. Then she instructed him to say to Mordecai, "All the king's officials and the people of the royal provinces know that for any man or woman who approaches the king in the inner court without being summoned the king has but one law: that they be put to death unless the king extends the gold scepter to them and spares their lives. But thirty days have passed since I was called to go to the king."
>
> —Esther 4:6–11 NIV

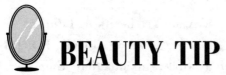

BEAUTY TIP

Accept it—God created a beautiful masterpiece in you.

MY FOUNDATION

MY FOUNDATION

BEAUTY 1-2-3

A FEW SIMPLE STEPS?

I read the disturbing news in one of my favorite women's magazines: "To take years off your age, refrain from putting eyeliner below the eyes."

Oh great! How old has this eyeliner made me look all these years? But another thought cheered me—if omitting eyeliner below my eyes was all it would take to look younger, I could handle this one. (And my morning makeup routine could be cut down by a whopping twenty seconds.)

I'm always game for trying new beauty methods. One sure way to get plenty of remedial help is to room with two Mary Kay beauty consultants at an overnight retreat. If you want immediate emergency beauty attention, just say, "I don't wash my face before I go to bed." It was like Indiana Jones swinging to my rescue with a James Bond, fully loaded, six-foot roll-out, quilted, pocketed, makeup travel pouch. I'd never owned that many beauty products in my entire lifetime! By the time my friends were through with me, I was cleansed, exfoliated, hydrated, revitalized, and moisturized.

Beauty plans are a dime a dozen. But knowing God's plan for our lives? It may not be as easy as a three-step beauty program or rooming with two beauty consultants. And you might be thinking, *I'd do God's plan if I just knew what it was.* So since you mentioned it, here are three ways to get started:

First, when we have a relationship with God, we have his Holy Spirit within us to guide us, to teach us, and to give us wisdom. Jesus said, "**But the Helper, the Holy Spirit, whom the Father will send in My name, He will teach you all things, and bring to your remembrance all that I said to you**" and "**But when He, the Spirit of truth, comes, He will guide you into all the truth**" (John 14:26; 16:13 NASB).

Second, we have the Bible for our source of unfaltering guidance. It gives us a picture of God. It shows God's parameters of godly living and instruction in what pleases him. **"All Scripture is God-breathed and is useful for teaching, rebuking, correcting and training in righteousness, so that the man [or woman!] of God may be thoroughly equipped for every good work"** (2 Timothy 3:16–17 NIV84).

Third, we have the awesome privilege of prayer—communication with the one who holds the plans to our lives. **"If any of you lacks wisdom, you should ask God, who gives generously to all without finding fault, and it will be given to you"** (James 1:5 NIV).

For many years I wondered what James meant when he said God would give us wisdom "without finding fault." But one day I simply thought about the words. God showed me that, when I ask for wisdom, he won't point an accusing finger at me and say, "Karen, I can't believe you're asking me this again! How many times do I have to tell you?"

Rather, God—in his love and through his Spirit and written Word—promises to show us and guide us in all knowledge. The apostle Peter reminds us, **"By his divine power, God has given us everything we need for living a godly life"** (2 Peter 1:3 NLT). We just have to ask, read his Word daily, and trust his Spirit for what we need.

THE ESTHER FACTOR

For sure Esther had a beauty plan, and it wasn't just 1-2-3. It was one to twelve—twelve months of cleansing oils, cosmetics, and perfumes. I think my Mary Kay friends would be jealous.

You might be thinking, *I'm not certain, but I'd sure like to see if twelve months of spa treatments would help my obedience.* But do we really think her spa treatments washed away Esther's fears about moving away from cousin Mordecai? Did all the pampering calm her as she was called upon to become the wife to a man of a different nationality and faith? Was it her apparently stunning beauty that helped her through the difficult events of her life?

Rather, I think it had more to do with her relationship with her God. Her cousin Mordecai was a Jew in the line of Benjamin. He was also a scribe who sat often at the king's gate, probably holding a high civil service position. He even risked his life to expose a murder plot against King Xerxes by two of the king's officers.

So Esther (or Hadassah, her Jewish name) was raised by a devout Jewish family member. She was no doubt taught about the God of Abraham, Isaac, and Jacob, and she drew on that knowledge and faith in the God of her family.

If our friend Esther exercised her faith and prayed in difficult times, can't we do that or more? We have much more of God's written Word than she did. We have the Spirit to intercede and guide us when we pray.

We also have Esther as our example that those who seek God can experience great wisdom in every decision of life. And that wisdom gives us insight into God's plan for us. Knowing the plan is just the beginning, but it's where we start. Esther started with her knowledge of a powerful God, put one step in front of the other, and moved ahead with God. We can do the same!

Now the king was attracted to Esther more than to any of the other women, and she won his favor and approval more than any of the other virgins. So he set a royal crown on her head and made her queen instead of Vashti. And the king gave a great banquet, Esther's banquet, for all his nobles and officials. He proclaimed a holiday throughout the provinces and distributed gifts with royal liberality.

—Esther 2:17–18 NIV

BEAUTY TIP

God's Spirit, God's Word, and prayer—your obedience beauty plan.

MY FOUNDATION

DAY 5

MY FOUNDATION

DON'T SLOUGH OFF

JUST GIT 'ER DONE!

Bridesmaids today have it tough. When I was a bridesmaid many years ago, all that was required was to throw a small bridal shower, buy a pair of white heels, show up at dressing time, and look adoringly at the bride as she walked down the aisle on her big day.

Now bridesmaids sometimes have to deal with Bridezilla. You know, that perfectionist bride who makes life difficult for everyone around her, demanding her own way, throwing tantrums if something wasn't done yesterday or the way she requested. And from what I gather, she doesn't shop at Walmart. I've heard this condition has an actual clinical diagnosis: acquired situational narcissism.

The name says it all.

Jesus talked about bridesmaids. Ten of them, to be specific, sometimes referred to as the ten virgins. Their responsibility was to prepare the bride for the groom. I doubt they arranged manicures for everyone or bachelorette parties to Vegas. All Jesus said is that they took lamps and went to meet the groom. Five of them were smart and took oil to replenish their lamps. The other five, well, not so smart. They went without backup fuel. And sure enough, when the groom's pending arrival was announced, the foolish ones had empty lamps—no oil. The only help the prepared bridesmaids offered was, **"Go to those who sell oil and buy some for yourselves"** (Matthew 25: 9 NIV). But when the foolish bridesmaids went to get what they should have already had, the groom came.

There must be hundreds of interpretations of this parable. But one bottom-line truth seems apparent—five girls weren't ready. They didn't do what they should have done. Why? Maybe they were too busy getting their own nails and hair done. Maybe they got caught up in all the other details. Or maybe they just procrastinated and didn't get to the oil store beforehand. Whatever the reason, Jesus said they were foolish because they weren't prepared for the big event.

We don't have literal weddings to prepare for every day; but the greatest wedding of all time will culminate when Jesus, the bridegroom, comes for his bride, the church—those of us who follow Jesus and have asked him to be Lord of our lives. We need to be prepared for the big day.

Our preparation is in the form of obeying God. It's that plan thing again!

However, some days I wouldn't be prepared if he showed up. Why do I procrastinate and fail to do what God wants? Sometimes I get self-centered (narcissistic, ouch!) and put my needs, wants, and agenda before God's plan. Other times, I get overwhelmed and sidetracked with life and "stuff" around me—"stuff" that really doesn't matter. Things that are not even on God's radar screen.

But the greatest reason I put off doing what I know God wants me to do is fear. Fear I might not be good enough to do what God wants. Fear of what others will think of me. Fear that I'll try, fail, and look foolish.

Then I remind myself that Jesus didn't call the bridesmaids foolish because they tried and failed. They were foolish because they didn't even try to do what they were supposed to. They simply did not prepare.

THE ESTHER FACTOR

Esther had twelve months to prepare to meet her potential future husband. And that wasn't twelve months of finding a photographer, hiring a cake decorator, or narrowing down the guest list. Oh no, that was twelve months of pampering herself with oils, cosmetics, and fragrances.

It sounds great to us, but I wonder whether she thought it was so wonderful. We think of our spa visits—ones that we bask in voluntarily because we've had a bad day. But Esther was there by someone else's mandate. She probably had no choice when the king's officials knocked on Mordecai's door to escort her away. And quite possibly she didn't have time to prepare for her new venture. So maybe, at best, Esther's beauty treatments seemed a consolation prize for being in unfamiliar surroundings and the possibility of having the king of Persia reject her because she wasn't exactly what he was looking for. What a way to make a girl's day!

Esther appears to have accepted the plan put before her and gone ahead to just get it done! At the palace she cooperated with the beauty regimen. She listened to wise counsel on what she should take when she went to see the king. Then later on she confronted a life-threatening situation—yes, with some fear, but she did it.

What if Esther had believed she wasn't good enough and went to the king believing she was a beauty-queen dropout? What if she hadn't prepared herself beforehand with fasting and prayer? What if she had decided to wait a few months before exposing an evil murder plan? Quite possibly many Jews would have lost their lives if she hadn't been a bold queen who acted when she needed to.

Esther didn't make excuses. She refused to refuse the plans that were put before her. She prepared herself with prayer and forged ahead with faith in God and help from those around her.

"Bring Haman at once," the king said, "so that we may do what Esther asks."

So the king and Haman went to the banquet Esther had prepared. As they were drinking wine, the king again asked Esther, "Now what is your petition? It will be given you. And what is your request? Even up to half the kingdom, it will be granted."

Esther replied, "My petition and my request is this: If the king regards me with favor and if it pleases the king to grant my petition and fulfill my request, let the king and Haman come tomorrow to the banquet I will prepare for them. Then I will answer the king's question."

—Esther 5:5–8 NIV

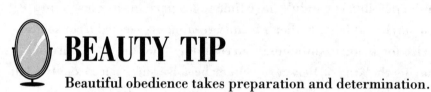

BEAUTY TIP

Beautiful obedience takes preparation and determination.

MY FOUNDATION

MY FOUNDATION

THE MOST IMPORTANT JOB

MINE!

In September 2010 an Australian emcee prepared to pronounce the winner and crown Australia's Next Top Model. Beside her stood the two remaining beautiful models in front of TV cameras and an audience of thousands. When the emcee announced the winner, the two contestants did what all beauty contestants do—they hugged, cried in disbelief, and congratulated each other. Then the winner began her acceptance speech.

What happened next was worse than a bad perm by a new hairstylist just before your class reunion. Amid the joyous commotion beside her, the emcee broke in. "I'm so sorry . . ." Silence filled the air as all eyes darted to the distressed announcer. "I don't know what to say. I'm feeling a bit sick about this, but . . ." Then she proceeded to inform the audience and contestants that she had announced the wrong winner![1]

More silence with dazed and confused looks. Everyone was probably wondering, *Was this covered in the Beauty Pageant Handbook? Who is supposed to do what after something like this?"* However, over the emcee's repeated apologies, the not-really-winner graciously turned and congratulated the real winner. The new real winner sputtered out a two-sentence acceptance speech and turned to walk the runway.

Have you ever felt second best? Maybe deep in the crevasses of your heart, you think you might have some potential—that you could accomplish something. But it seems like someone other than you always gets to walk down the runway, and you declare everyone else the winner instead of you.

We seem to be queens at giving up our crowns, thinking that someone else is more important, more talented, or more capable than we are. We begin to categorize whose lives, ministries, or service roles are more significant. We look at others' accomplishments, educational degrees, and, yes, even dress sizes and think their lives are more noteworthy than ours.

Jesus blew that theory when he taught about the parable of the talents (Matthew 25:14–30). As a master returned from a trip, he commended each servant who invested the money he had given them before his departure. One servant had earned four talents for the master and another earned ten. But he told them both, "**Well done, good and faithful servant! You have been faithful with a few things; I will put you in charge of many things. Come and share your master's happiness!**" (v. 23).

So when the master, who in this case represented God, looked at his servants' lives, he didn't see quantity. He saw faithfulness.

I have come to the brilliant conclusion that there will always be others who get more notoriety and public exposure and have a longer list of accomplishments than I do. But God doesn't consider the plans for one of his children more important than his plans for someone else. He is looking for faithfulness to what he called me to do. Working at God's plan to the best of my ability in cooperation with his Holy Spirit is what's important.

God isn't keeping score. He's looking for those who will be fully committed to play on his team, no matter the position.

THE ESTHER FACTOR

If anyone could feel like second best, it might have been Esther. She followed a very lovely predecessor, Queen Vashti, the First Lady of Persia. In fact, she was so lovely that King Xerxes commanded her to display her beautiful little face and lovely crown at his banquet. However, she refused. It was this refusal that led to all the hullabaloo to take her crown and search for another queen.

So Esther was coming in as a replacement. She could very easily have been tempted to wonder whether the king would compare her to Queen Vashti. Was she as pretty? Was she poised and proper like a queen should be? Would the king consider her second best?

It's ironic to think about because most of us look at Esther's life and think, *Oh, I'll never do anything as important as her. After all, she has a book in the Bible named after her.*

Esther was where she was because God chose her to do a specific job. He had looked down through time and observed a plot would be devised against his exiled chosen people by an arrogant kingdom official. He also saw a young Jewish orphan and chose to put her in place to combat this deceitful ploy. We too are given our life plans by God because he needs some tasks accomplished.

I need to stop spending time evaluating whether my name will appear at the top of some heavenly corporate organizational chart, as if some positions are more weighty than others. God simply has a design for his universe, and we are joint heirs working with others to glorify him and accomplish his purposes.

And by the way, our obedience is not measured by the size of the task. Sometimes the most challenging yet God-honoring obedience is shown in our everyday lives, the seemingly little decisions we make each day. The way we talk to our spouses. How we treat others. The respect we give to other drivers on the highway. Our attitude toward the grumpy waitress. Our compassion to the needy. These choices show whether we are really following God.

Esther accomplished a big task in our eyes. But whatever we do in obedience to God is a big one in his book.

On the seventh day, when King Xerxes was in high spirits from wine, he commanded the seven eunuchs who served him—Mehuman, Biztha, Harbona, Bigtha, Abagtha, Zethar and Karkas—to bring before him Queen Vashti, wearing her royal crown, in order to display her beauty to the people and nobles, for she was lovely to look at. But when the attendants delivered the king's command, Queen Vashti refused to come. Then the king became furious and burned with anger. . . .

"Then Memukan replied in the presence of the king and the nobles, "Queen Vashti has done wrong, not only against the king but also against all the nobles and the peoples of all the provinces of King Xerxes. . . .

"Therefore, if it pleases the king, let him issue a royal decree and let it be written in the laws of Persia and Media, which cannot be repealed, that Vashti is never again to enter the presence of King Xerxes. Also let the king give her royal position to someone else who is better than she."

—Esther 1:10–12, 16, 19 NIV

BEAUTY TIP

You may not save an entire nation from destruction, but God's plan for your life is important to *him*.

MY FOUNDATION

MY FOUNDATION

ARE YOU A SPRING OR A WINTER?

GOD'S CHANGING SEASONS

Did you know that the colors we wear in clothes and makeup can attract love, increase powers, restore energy, and help us make a lasting impression on the world? I read this in an article about color palettes named after seasons, and I thought, *Really? That's all it takes? And to think I've been exercising, reading books on how to schmooze my husband, and listening to motivational speakers. Apparently, all I had to do was change my shirt and eye shadow.*

I read further. The article described seasons, not the kind of seasons we learned about in kindergarten during calendar time but the concept that all of us fit into either a spring, summer, fall, or winter color palette. And it's not determined by whether our favorite holiday is Christmas or the Fourth of July. It's based on our skin tones and hair and eye colors. For me, calendar time seemed much more doable and sensible. Trying to determine what beauty season I fit in left me feeling like a climate-confused beauty schizophrenic.

I am, however, familiar with the other seasons of our lives such as the spring of our young, carefree school days and the summer of entering the workplace and, possibly, marriage and family. Fall is colorful with learning about AARP, deciding on a retirement date, and being an empty nester. And, finally, the golden days of winter, when, hopefully, we can do what we want, when we want, even if that means wearing no makeup and eating popcorn for breakfast. Our lives change, and I believe God's plan moves us through stages of life, ministry, and service.

I remember a distinct change of season in my life. Having been at home with the kids for a number of years, I began a new season working outside the home. The job became a real challenge. I was employed doing tasks I didn't feel qualified for, things I wasn't sure I had a passion for, and duties I never thought I would be performing.

Two weeks on the job and I was miserable. I came home some nights and cried. I complained to my husband and anyone who dared ask, "How's your job?" I lashed out at God, "If I had to get a job, would it have been such a big deal to get me something I actually liked?" Other days I questioned God through tears, "What in the world am I doing here?"

Over the next few months, as I grew more frustrated and discontented, I began sensing something different. I didn't want to admit it at first, but it seemed that, for some unknown crazy reason, I was exactly where God wanted me to be. As God softened my heart to that idea, I began to accept my season of life.

One day, driving home after a particularly draining day at work, a song came on the radio. The words reminded me that God wasn't finished with me yet. It was an old cliché put to a new melody, but its truth rang loud in my heart that afternoon. I felt God telling me I wouldn't be at this job forever. Someday I would be in another season, doing the things that I thought more aligned with my purpose here on this earth. But, for now, this is where God had me.

King Solomon reminds us, **"There is a time for everything, and a season for every activity under heaven"** (Ecclesiastes 3:1 NIV84). What season are you in? Are you struggling? Have you poured out all your misgivings to God and then allowed him to soften your heart?

You might be right where God wants you. Go with the plan and see what God can do through you.

THE ESTHER FACTOR

Remember Esther's cousin Mordecai? From what we know about him, he also transitioned through several seasons of life.

First, he was part of an exiled nation living in a foreign land—maybe not the best season of life. At some point, however, he found his way to being a scribe and hanging out at the king's gate. This was a slight shift through the seasons, maybe an upgrade. It was during his tenure at the palace gate that he found out about an assassination plot by two of the king's officers. He reported the scheme, the officers ended up hanged, and eventually Mordecai was honored throughout the city as a hero.

Another season arrived for Mordecai after he requested the newly elected Queen Esther to expose another plot—this time aimed at killing all the Jewish people living in the land. He sent Esther a message that Haman, the highest-ranking kingdom official, had tricked King Xerxes into signing a decree that would allow the murder of all the Jews on a certain day.

Esther bravely informed the king, a new decree was signed to save the Jews, and (*spoiler alert!*) Mordecai was honored again and consequently given Haman's high place of authority in the land.

Mordecai endured plenty of drama and danger throughout these seasons. From a foreigner, to a respected citizen, to a king's highly honored official, Mordecai stayed true to his God. The seasons played out, and by not swerving in his allegiance to God, Mordecai enjoyed the final season of his life in prosperity.

But most important of all, Mordecai's obedience to God caused many in the land to sit up and take notice of the God of the Jews. God was honored through the faithful efforts of Mordecai during all the seasons of his life.

What a great legacy we can leave—that many would look at our lives, see our faithfulness to God through all our seasons, and then be challenged to follow our God!

When the virgins were assembled a second time, Mordecai was sitting at the king's gate. But Esther had kept secret her family background and nationality just as Mordecai had told her to do, for she continued to follow Mordecai's instructions as she had done when he was bringing her up.

During the time Mordecai was sitting at the king's gate, Bigthana and Teresh, two of the king's officers who guarded the doorway, became angry and conspired to assassinate King Xerxes. But Mordecai found out about the plot and told Queen Esther, who in turn reported it to the king, giving credit to Mordecai. And when the report was investigated and found to be true, the two officials were hanged on gallows. All this was recorded in the book of the annals in the presence of the king.

—Esther 2:19–23 NIV

BEAUTY TIP

Obedience through our changing seasons helps us leave a beautiful legacy.

MY FOUNDATION

MY FOUNDATION

TAKE THIS JOB AND LOVE IT!

CONTENTMENT, NOT COMPARISON

Years ago I handed my hairstylist a photo of a beautiful model. "I want this haircut," I said.

She looked at the photo, glanced at me and then back at the photo, and proceeded to choose her words very carefully. "You know," she said with a slight grin, "Many times a woman will say she wants her hair in a certain style when in reality she wants to look like the woman herself."

I'm still not sure why she said that to me. The nerve!

OK, I'll admit it. More than once I've looked at someone else and thought, *Oh, if I just had her legs . . . or her waist . . . or her upper arms without wings* (as my daughter lovingly calls them). But I have to admit, most of the time I have hair envy. Everyone else's hair minds so well.

At times I'm tempted to think the same things about God's plan for my life. I look at my friends' lives and think, *Why can't I sing like Mary, God? I could really bless people.* Or, *If only I had Susie's servant heart. Think of the people I could help.* And, *Lord, why can't I have a confident personality like Kim? I could tell the whole world about you.*

It's one thing to be inspired by those around us and quite another to let God's plan and will for *their* lives distract us from running our own God-given race. The writer of Hebrews refers to that race: **"Therefore . . . let us throw off everything that hinders and the sin that so easily entangles, and let us run with perseverance the race marked out for us"** (Hebrews 12:1 NIV84).

That little two-letter word *us* makes a big difference. Or to personalize it: me. I should run the race marked out for *me*.

Imagine running the 400-yard dash. (I'm out of breath already.) The gun goes off, and I sprint down the track. But I suddenly decide I like the lane next to me better. *I'll just run over here*, I think, as I take over my opponent's lane. Then my feet entangle with hers, and both of us tumble headlong, nose first. I'm thinking skinned knees, bloody elbows, and scraped hands—not to mention what it would do to my hair! Girls, this is not a pretty picture.

The obsession of *if only!* If only I had her personality, her bank account, or her job, then I could be more content to live a godly life. If only I had a husband like hers or compliant kids like hers, then I'd have the support I need to follow God. Thoughts like this can hinder our race, slow us down, and eventually entangle us in mind games counterproductive to living the plan God has for us. I've learned I can run the race marked out for me, even on a bad-hair day, and even if I can't do it exactly like someone else.

God made each of us with our own specific life plans. God has made us in such a way that we can carry out his purposes for our lives. I'm not suggesting we can't work on some undesirable character trait or color our hair or that we shouldn't work to earn more money. But there has to be an inner contentment with how God has made us, our positions in life, and the places where he's called us to serve.

The Esther Factor

Do you think Queen Esther ever wanted someone else's job? Or life? Do you think she ever thought, *This isn't exactly the life I thought I signed up for?* I mean, one day she is happily tending house at cousin Mordecai's, the next minute she's whisked off to the Miss Persia Beauty Pageant, only to find out later she's entered into *Mission Impossible*.

Do you suppose she thought, *Oh, why can't I just be back home tending the garden like Rebekah?* Or, *Why did I have to be an orphan? Why couldn't I have two parents like Shiprah?* Or maybe, *Doggone that Queen Vashti! If she'd obeyed in the first place, I wouldn't be here!*

We really don't know for sure whether Esther played the comparison game or not. But there is an interesting thing she did while in the king's harem. Each girl from the harem had the opportunity to take whatever she wanted from the palace when it was her turn to visit the king. However, Scripture makes special note that Esther was content with taking only what Hegai, the king's attendant in charge of the harem, suggested. For whatever reason, Esther chose to take his advice, no matter what the other girls were doing. Her contentment with doing this ended in her being crowned the next queen.

Esther appears not to have been so concerned with what was going on around her. Rather, she was open to good counsel. Maybe there is some validity in running our own races, making our own choices, and doing what we need to do instead of trying to be like someone else. Esther ran the race marked out for her.

So let's let our beauty shine, by running our own races and doing what God puts before us!

> And this is how [each young virgin] would go to the king:
> Anything she wanted was given her to take with her from
> the harem to the king's palace. In the evening she would

go there and in the morning return to another part of
the harem to the care of Shaashgaz, the king's eunuch
in charge of the concubines. She would not return to the
king unless he was pleased with her and summoned her by
name.

When the turn came for Esther . . . to go to the king,
she asked for nothing other than what Hegai, the king's
eunuch who was in charge of the harem, suggested. And
Esther won the favor of everyone who saw her.

—Esther 2:13–15 NIV

BEAUTY TIP

God loves it when you embrace his plan for your life and
run with it.

MY FOUNDATION

PART 2

THE PROBLEMS

THE GRAND ILLUSION

WAS IT THE MIRRORS?

As a child, I occasionally heard about a celebrity having a face-lift or a tummy tuck. Face-lift? Tummy tuck? I couldn't imagine this. To where does one lift her face? And I could tuck my own tummy if you'd tell me where to hide it!

Today it seems you are the exception if you haven't had cosmetic surgery. From 1997–2007, cosmetic surgeries rose a mere 457 percent, according to the American Society for Aesthetic Plastic Surgery. And what are we getting surgery for? Certainly not life-threatening situations, but popular procedures such as liposuction, breast augmentation, eyelid surgery, and some nonsurgical procedures such as Botox injections and laser hair removal!

The thought seems to be that, plastic surgery will solve all your beauty problems. Just get some surgery and everything will be OK!

Not one to miss out on the latest fads, I thought I should check into this. So one afternoon I took a serious look at my body in a full-length mirror—despite my recent Pringles, dark chocolate, and Diet Coke. Starting with a safe place, I studied my face. I placed three fingers on each side of my eyes and pulled slightly upward and back—the only conceivable destination I could think to lift my face.

Hmm. Yes, it brought back memories of my younger years—my look when my mom pulled my pigtails too tight.

One dermatologist says she is treating more patients in their twenties and thirties with "preventative Botox."[2] They want injections to keep the problem wrinkles from happening in the first place. It gives a new twist to the term *preventative healthcare*!

I don't know about you, but to me this is just weird. To think we will never look old? Wouldn't it be strange to stroll through a nursing home where everyone looks thirty?

I rather doubt we can prevent all wrinkles and signs of aging—just like we cannot prevent problems in other areas of our live. But sometimes we mistakenly believe the illusion that if we just follow Jesus, everything will be OK.

The apostle Peter burst that bubble when he warned first-century believers, **"Dear friends, do not be surprised at the painful trial you are suffering, as though something strange were happening to you. But rejoice that you participate in the sufferings of Christ, so that you may be overjoyed when his glory is revealed. If you are insulted because of the name of Christ, you are blessed, for the Spirit of glory and of God rests on you"** (1 Peter 4:12–14 NIV84).

We know how to make food salt-free, fat-free, and gluten-free. We can make cosmetics oil-free, streak-free, and fragrance-free. However, no one has figured out how to make life trouble-free. So maybe we should just accept the fact that we will have problems.

THE ESTHER FACTOR

Beautiful Esther had her share of tough times. Her people had been taken captive and lived as exiles in a foreign land. Then her parents died while she was still young.

But shortly thereafter, Esther found herself transferred to the king's palace. King Xerxes was looking for a new queen, and because of her beauty, Esther was chosen to enter the beauty contest to become the new and improved First Lady.

At first, this seemed like an upgrade—moving from the neighborhood of exiles to the citadel of Susa. (By the way, a citadel is like a stronghold or fortified city. So consider this a move to the first gated community.) The icing on the cake was special food and beauty treatments. Esther even placed in the semifinals of the Mrs. Persia pageant. Hegai, the eunuch in charge of the beauty contestants, was pleased with Esther and moved her to the best quarters of the palace. She went on to finally win the crown.

Reading just that far in her story, we might be tempted to believe the illusion that Esther's life was smooth and problem-free, that everything was going to be OK. But Esther had no idea what was about to happen. Haman, a high-ranking official in her new home, became disgruntled at her cousin Mordecai. Mordecai refused to bow in Haman's presence, even though the king had commanded everyone to do so as Haman passed.

Rage filled Haman's heart, and he embarked on a passionate quest to kill Mordecai and the rest of the Jews. Haman rigged some accusations against the Jewish people and asked the king's permission to kill the supposed infidels. When Esther found out about the plot to exterminate her people, she was faced with some heart-wrenching, life-threatening decisions.

All the beauty treatments in the world, a luxurious life in a palace, and coming from a devout Jewish family didn't immunize Esther from the difficulties that lay ahead. Esther's life was far from problem-free.

When Haman saw that Mordecai would not kneel down or pay him honor, he was enraged. Yet having learned who Mordecai's people were, he scorned the idea of killing only Mordecai. Instead Haman looked for a way to destroy all Mordecai's people, the Jews, throughout the whole kingdom of Xerxes.

—Esther 3:5–6 NIV

 # BEAUTY TIP

It's no illusion—even on our journey of following God, we will have problems.

MY FOUNDATION

MY FOUNDATION

CONCEALERS

THE NAME SAYS IT ALL

J en, do you have some concealer?" I asked my daughter-in-law. I had stayed overnight with her and my son to help them get settled in their new house. "These dark circles under my eyes are atrocious!" I stared in dismay at the mirror.

She opened the bathroom cabinet and pulled out a tote with beauty products. She dug through the box and found a bottle. "Here. Try this."

I studied the bottle in my hand. "I've never used concealer before," I said.

Jen whisked off to do something else. She should have stayed. What happened next was bad news.

Oh, I did mention I'd never used this type of product before, didn't I? I submit ignorance as my defense. I dabbed a little of the cream under my eyes, but it didn't seem to blend in with the rest of my face. So I did what anyone with my level of beauty intelligence would do: I covered my whole face with concealer.

Now, if one should *happen* to rub concealer all over her face, shouldn't her face be, um, concealed? But not mine. At my first check in the mirror, I thought, *This isn't going on so well. Maybe I better rub it in more.* I rubbed, and rubbed, and rubbed. Something told me I shouldn't have done that. (Ever get those feelings?) You've heard the phrase "white as a ghost"? I looked like I was ready for Halloween. What was meant to cover up only magnified the problem.

Cover-ups in areas other than cosmetics also have a way of backfiring and magnifying unfortunate events. Has anyone ever concealed something from you? And I'm not talking about her face. Maybe someone you considered a friend said hurtful things behind your back? Or a coworker tried to cover up her misdeeds in the office and asked you not to report her? Or an adult child continued law-breaking activities and expected family support? Maybe a spouse was dishonest about finances or your relationship?

Face it: other people cause all kinds of trouble in all kinds of ways. And while "I don't deserve this" may be the absolute truth in the situation, adopting a victim mentality seldom helps but leads to self-pity, selfishness, and all those other *self* attitudes.

When we're hurt, we need to choose between forgiveness or exposure. Jesus was clear that forgiveness toward others is related to the forgiveness of our own sins: **"But if you do not forgive men their sins, your Father will not forgive your sins"** (Matthew 6:15, NIV84).

You might say, "Yeah, but I can't forgive him" or "You don't know what she did to me."

I don't, but God does. And he's the one who gave us the forgiveness factor. He knew forgiveness would put our hearts at peace again and that he can work more effectively through us when we're not harboring bitterness.

Other situations might need exposure, confronting our offenders in Christian love and firmness. But this should always involve prayer and leading by the Holy Spirit. This may be a time to get good, godly counsel from a pastor or close Christian sister.

People are going to hurt us. But our responses make the difference in whether we continue to live in beauty or not.

THE ESTHER FACTOR

We've heard about the apostle Paul and his thorn in the flesh. Esther had her thorn in the flesh too. His name was Haman. If you'll remember, he was one of King Xerxes's highest officials.

As Esther became familiar with palace life, she became acquainted with Haman. I mean, how could she not? He had been ranked above all the other kingdom officials. He owned vast wealth. He had a large family. And the king had commanded that everyone bow when Haman passed by. He was hard to miss.

But Haman got his knickers in a wad because Mordecai would not bow down to him as the king had ordered. Haman would not rest until he got rid of Mordecai—and all the rest of the Jews.

Haman devised a scheme to trick the king. At a secret meeting, Haman told the king there were some people living in the land who did not follow the Persian law and customs. There was a certain amount of truth to this statement. The people Haman had on his devious little mind were the Jews. They followed God's law and their own customs, but they certainly had no intent to overthrow the government!

However, as Haman continued to cunningly omit the identification of these people, he suggested that the king should not tolerate them—but kill them. Haman promised the king a ten thousand–talent donation to the royal treasury. With hardly a blink, the king signed a decree as Haman requested. "And, oh, by the way," the king added, "you can keep the money."

Word traveled fast in Persia. And Mordecai heard of the plot as the murder edict was issued. He sent Esther word through a messenger about the deceit and murder and asked her to do the impossible: approach the king and expose the lies. But Esther and Mordecai both knew that to do so could mean Esther's death.

So what do you do with a thorn like Haman? His utter contempt for her cousin Mordecai and then his murder plan were enough to gray her hair and develop premature wrinkles, not to mention giving her sleepless nights. Was her response forgiveness or exposure?

Because of the extreme danger and outright evil of the situation, Esther chose to expose the plan. I doubt it was an easy decision. Making the choice between forgiveness and confrontation is hard when others are causing us trouble. But Esther shows us it's not impossible. The key is that she moved forward with much prayer and fasting.

> Then Haman said to King Xerxes, "There is a certain people dispersed among the peoples in all the provinces of your kingdom who keep themselves separate. Their customs are different from those of all other people, and they do not obey the king's laws; it is not in the king's best interest to tolerate them. If it pleases the king, let a decree be issued to destroy them, and I will give ten thousand talents of silver to the king's administrators for the royal treasury."
>
> So the king took his signet ring from his finger and gave it to Haman son of Hammedatha, the Agagite, the enemy of the Jews. "Keep the money," the king said to Haman, "and do with the people as you please."
>
> —Esther 3:8–11 NIV

BEAUTY TIP

Depend on God to help with the concealers and evildoers along your journey.

MY FOUNDATION

MY FOUNDATION

A WRINKLE IN TIME

LIFE IN THESE TIMES

What are those?" I shrieked as I looked in the mirror. I ran my fingers across my cheeks. Whatever they were smoothed themselves out momentarily, only to return when I stopped pulling on my face. Soon it was evident: those whatevers were wrinkles.

"Where did you come from?" I squinted and asked, as if they would answer. I'm sure there is a scientific explanation for how sagging begins and wrinkles take up residence on our bodies. But surely I was too young for this!

Some months later, sitting in the waiting room at my doctor's office, I thought I'd found the cure to those nasty facial crinkles. On the wall hung a whiteboard with the heading, "Wine and Wrinkles." Below the title were bullet points:

- Better than Botox.
- Softens wrinkles.
- Improves muscle tone.
- Lifts sagging eyelids.
- Decreases puffiness and bags under eyes.
- Reduces double chins (my favorite).

The doctor walked by. I pointed to the board and said, "So, do you ingest it or rub it on your face?"

He seemed puzzled.

"The wine," I said, motioning at the board again. "Do you drink it or rub it on your face?"

He chuckled. "Oh, neither. They had a wine sampling party here last night while they discussed acupuncture facelift. Acupuncture is great for wrinkles and sagging."

Part of me was relieved. I don't drink wine, and I didn't know how to convince myself to visit a liquor store in quest of wrinkle reducing. On the other hand, I wasn't too keen on trying the acupuncture facelift. Maybe in time . . .

The problems we encounter in life—and those doggone wrinkles—seem to just show up, don't they? One day we're a contented, pretty little face, and the next day something much worse than wrinkles comes along. A situation threatens our peace and joy and possibly even tries to interrupt us on our journey of following God. Maybe it's a bad medical report, a job layoff, the premature death of a loved one.

As we wonder why these problems come, it's important to remember where we came from. In the beginning, God created a perfect world, without disease, death, or conflict. Mankind quickly took care of that by sinning. In Genesis 3, we read that after Adam and Eve ate the prohibited fruit, **"the eyes of both of them were opened, and they realized they were naked"** (v. 7 NIV).

Eve wasn't stressed simply because she wasn't going to look good in fig leaves. She didn't even know the word *naked* until she disobeyed God and saw her sin. Disobedience brought sin into our world, and it's never left. After sin, God doled out the consequences. And it is clear in Genesis 3 that our lives on planet Earth would no longer be perfect.

So some of our struggles in life are going to come just because we live in an imperfect world. We need to remember, though, that God doesn't leave us alone. Later we will talk about God's power that helps us through life, even in the midst of struggles. In the meantime, refuse to let those struggles affect your walk with God. Because, after all, just like wrinkles, those struggles are temporary.

The Esther Factor

Esther could have adopted the victim mentality. She could have thought, I *didn't do anything to deserve living in this foreign country. And I certainly didn't deserve to be an orphan!*

Esther's people had been taken into captivity because of their disobedience to God. So here was Esther, a Jew, living in Persia as a result of the sin around her. And her parents died. Add those two unfortunate events, and you have the recipe for a potentially bitter or discouraged young lady.

But we never get that impression of Esther from Scripture. The first we read of her, she is being taken off to the palace, probably not of her own accord, as a possible replacement for the queen. This could be added to her I-don't-deserve-this list also. But it seems Esther made the best of it and followed the counsel of those in charge of her, and she ended up First Lady of Persia.

So what was her secret to pushing through when all these things were threatening to push her down? Simple—Esther knew her God. She did not give in to despair when everything around her seemed to fall apart or wasn't going the way she would have liked. Instead, she faced each next event with confidence that her God was going to take care of her. She made decisions, planned courses of action, and depended on God to work it all out.

Was she confident all the time? Did she feel secure when her parents died? Did she feel safe and sound as she was being taken by the king's officials away from cousin Mordecai? Maybe. Maybe not. But trials have a way of building confidence in our powerful God as we depend on him and see him work.

Just ask Esther.

> Now there was in the citadel of Susa a Jew of the tribe
> of Benjamin, named Mordecai son of Jair, the son of
> Shimei, the son of Kish, who had been carried into exile
> from Jerusalem by Nebuchadnezzar king of Babylon,

among those taken captive with Jehoiachin king of Judah.
Mordecai had a cousin named Hadassah, whom he had
brought up because she had neither father nor mother.
This young woman, who was also known as Esther, had a
lovely figure and was beautiful. Mordecai had taken her as
his own daughter when her father and mother died.

—Esther 2:5–7 NIV

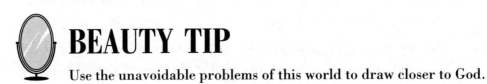

BEAUTY TIP

Use the unavoidable problems of this world to draw closer to God.

MY FOUNDATION

MY FOUNDATION

Wasn't Me! Or Was It?

I munched on the last bite of my lunch, and almost gloated: grilled chicken strips wrapped in lettuce leaves and a low-carb tortilla. Foregoing the chips, I smugly complemented my low-calorie, healthy lunch with carrot sticks on the side and a cool glass of water. Sign me up for the Healthy Eaters Rewards Club.

Putting my plate in the dishwasher, I thought, *I need just a little sweet to top off this meal.* I checked the fridge. Nothing there. Freezer? Ah, yes, just what I need—a little chocolate. That's when I fell off the wagon. My one dip of chocolate ice cream turned into two, and before you could say, "Chocolate is a girl's best friend," I had that frozen confection laden with Oreo crumbles and smothered in chocolate syrup.

I didn't mean to. I really didn't! Blame it on arrogance. All I could think was, *I'm so good . . . just a little won't hurt!* The operative word was *little*, and I didn't comply. I was disturbed at the bloated feeling I had later—and the residual guilty feelings. I had no one to blame but myself.

Yep, like we've talked the past few days, sometimes problems come from the sin in this world and sometimes they come from other people. But sometimes we cause our own problems! And if we're still talking food, I've experienced a number of food-induced problems of my own making, from weight increases to low energy, from joint pain to larger jeans.

However, we know food isn't our only problem, and probably not our biggest. When I choose to use an uncontrolled tongue, I hurt relationships. If I continue to spend more money than I make, I have bills I can't pay and creditors looking for me. When I refuse to control my temper, others aren't too anxious to be around me. If I don't exercise, I risk heart disease and many other ailments.

But the problems run deeper than injured relationships, bills, or being sick. Those are simply signs of deeper heart issues. When I gossip, the source might be jealousy or bitterness. Uncontrolled spending of money might indicate discontent or an addiction to materialism.

Do you see the point here? When I cause myself problems, the problems are the symptoms. I need to look deeper to correct my heart. I'd like to submit a theory that has proven true time and again in my own life: I believe that every sin has pride at its root. Check out the middle letter of *pride*.

If I'm jealous, my pride is being threatened. If I want more and more "stuff," it's either to show off, fill a void in my life, or feel important. If I lash out at my husband or am uncompassionate or selfish, I certainly am not thinking of him. I have me on my mind—my feelings, my convenience, my ego—and that is pride.

Do the test in your own life. Think of your last sin. (Time's up— doesn't take long, huh?) How did the sin show itself? What was your emotion at the time? And why do you think you felt that way? Was the problem you? And was pride involved?

Don't beat yourself up, though. Confess your sin and ask forgiveness. We may have brought it on ourselves, but 1 John 1:9 says, **"If we confess our sins, he is faithful and just and will forgive us our sins and purify us from all unrighteousness"** (NIV).

And forgiveness is much more satisfying than chocolate.

The Esther Factor

To say Haman was prideful is a bit like saying Angelina Jolie is cute. Haman certainly owned the corner on the market of pride. And Angie? Well, some might say she has her own corner.

We've already learned that King Xerxes had commanded those at the king's gate to bow when Haman approached. Maybe that was the start of Haman's arrogance. But it didn't help that he was prolific, wealthy, and in high authority. Credentials like that can lead one down the path of temptation, and Haman followed like a bloodhound on a fox chase. Ironically, his pride led to a rather humbling event. It reminds me of a warning from God, **"Pride goes before destruction, a haughty spirit before a fall" (Proverbs 16:18** NIV**).**

It all started when King Xerxes couldn't sleep one night, so he ordered that the diaries of his kingly reign be brought to him. As his attendants read some palace history, it was noted that a Jew named Mordecai had uncovered an assassination attempt on the king's life. When the king asked if Mordecai had been duly recognized, the attendants reported that nothing had been done.

Haman just happened to be entering the king's court at this time, and the king summoned him in. Xerxes sought Haman's input. He asked, "What should be done for the man the king delights to honor?"

Pride swelled in Haman's heart. The king had to be thinking about him! So Haman outlined the greatest plan of the century: honor this man with a royal robe, put him on a royal horse adorned with a royal crest, and have a royal official lead him through the city.

Oops! When the curtain opens again, we see Haman, as ordered by King Xerxes, parading Mordecai, his arch nemesis, through the city on a royal horse, with a royal crest, and wearing a royal robe. Haman went home royally humiliated.

Haman brought on his own embarrassment, and pride was the springboard. Too bad this wasn't the extent to which his pride got him in trouble. We'll learn more about that tomorrow.

When Haman entered, the king asked him, "What should be done for the man the king delights to honor?"

Now Haman thought to himself, "Who is there that the king would rather honor than me?" So he answered the king, "For the man the king delights to honor, have them bring a royal robe the king has worn and a horse the king has ridden, one with a royal crest placed on its head. Then let the robe and horse be entrusted to one of the king's most noble princes. Let them robe the man the king delights to honor, and lead him on the horse through the city streets, proclaiming before him, 'This is what is done for the man the king delights to honor!'"

"Go at once," the king commanded Haman. "Get the robe and the horse and do just as you have suggested for Mordecai the Jew, who sits at the king's gate. Do not neglect anything you have recommended."

So Haman got the robe and the horse. He robed Mordecai, and led him on horseback through the city streets, proclaiming before him, "This is what is done for the man the king delights to honor!"

Afterward Mordecai returned to the king's gate. But Haman rushed home, with his head covered in grief.

—Esther 6:6–12 NIV

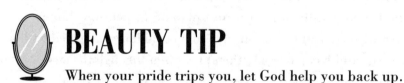

BEAUTY TIP

When your pride trips you, let God help you back up.

MY FOUNDATION

MY FOUNDATION

THE ONE THING
I CAN'T HAVE

IT'S NOT WORTH IT

"Try this straightening iron," my stylist said after she had crafted my new 'do. "It's top of the line. I love it." I clamped the iron onto a section of hair, and it glided down like hot fudge on the side of a double-scoop sundae.

"Wow, I want one of these," I said, trying not to sound too lustful. "Where can I get one?"

"You can buy them at the beauty supply store. But they're about eighty dollars."

She put the finishing touches on my hair. I glanced longingly at my new gotta-have beauty toy as I turned to leave. The feel of the iron still reverberated on every strand of my hair. I wasn't sure this was a good thing.

I drove home, my mind consumed with that doggone curling iron. I even felt frustration brewing. For Pete's sake, I came from back in the 1970s when we girls used a real iron to straighten our hair. We'd come a long way, baby, in beauty-appliance technology, and I wanted this state-of-the-art iron! Even though I knew I couldn't justify the purchase, every hair on my head yearned for its smooth, elegant touch.

Have you ever wanted something really bad? So much so that you got irritated because it was out of your budget, out of your reach, or simply out of the question? Did you focus on it until you became cynical, bitter, or even blamed God because he hadn't answered your prayer. Do I need to mention this isn't a good thing?

Usually the things we can't have but still want end up causing us problems. And usually the things what we want are more serious than beauty tools. We could want other significant material possessions. There could be relationships we want to be in, positions at work, or status among our circles of friends. Or maybe we want someone else to change, yet we know we have no control over him or her.

There are several issues here. First, sometimes we get to the point that we are more frustrated that we can't have it than we are with the fact that we don't have it! It's the difference in permission and possession. Bizarre as this seems, sometimes we just want to know we *can* have something, whether we actually get it or not. I'm not sure whether I've mentioned it— but this isn't a good thing.

The second problem with wanting a certain possession, status, or control is that once it consumes our thoughts and energies, God can't use us fully because, well, how do I say this . . . something else has taken first place in our lives. Whether it's a desire for something or the possession itself, anything more important to us than God is an idol.

Sometimes the lengths we go through to obtain something we really desire end up hurting others and even ourselves. If it's a job, position, or control we want, we may not care whose feelings get hurt or whose reputation gets marred in the process. We risk relationships and our character, and it doesn't reflect too well on our being Christians either

The bottom line here is that our ambition to do God's will should be our greatest desire in life. We can work at a smaller dress size if needed, we can spiff up our homes to make them more comfortable, and we can work hard to get a promotion. But if any of these is more important than pleasing God, it's an idol. And oh, did I mention that isn't a good thing?

THE ESTHER FACTOR

Haman had a hang-up about something he couldn't have. In fact, his hang-up was so bad it—well, hold on to those words for a moment. I don't want to ruin the surprise at the end of this story.

Let's start by going over again what Haman did have: the highest authority in the land, right under the king; wealth spilling from his money bags; a big family with many sons; the prestige of having everyone bow to him; two invitations to royal banquets at the palace; and the king's honor and trust.

So, what part of *content* didn't he understand?

One day at a gathering of his family and friends, Haman recounted all his fame, fortune, and family proliferation. Then after boasting about all this, he said, "But . . ." (Ever noticed how the word *but* can get us into trouble?)

Haman continued, "But all this gives me no satisfaction as long as I see that Jew Mordecai sitting at the king's gate." His hang-up was Mordecai and the fact that Mordecai would not bow in his presence. So forgetting everything he already had, he fixated on the one thing he didn't have.

Do you know people like this? People who, no matter how much good is in their lives, still find one thing they can't have, one thing to complain about, and one thing to make them discontented? The sad thing is that one thing of discontent can very well become the thing that destroys them.

What did it do to Haman? His hang-up got him hung up. After his childish outburst, Haman built some gallows intended for Mordecai. But what happened next was more embarrassing than being pulled over for speeding when you have a Christian bumper sticker on your car. Right after Esther exposed Haman's deceitful scheme to kill the Jews, the king ordered Haman hung on his own gallows. Haman's fixation on the one thing he didn't have eventually killed him.

Too bad that wasn't all the damage done. His sons ended up being hung too, and thousands of Persian soldiers sent to destroy the Jews were also killed. Haman's obsession with what he couldn't have had devastating consequences.

And that, my friends, is absolutely, most assuredly, not a good thing.

> Haman went out that day happy and in high spirits. But when he saw Mordecai at the king's gate and observed that he neither rose nor showed fear in his presence, he was filled with rage against Mordecai. Nevertheless, Haman restrained himself and went home.
>
> Calling together his friends and Zeresh, his wife, Haman boasted to them about his vast wealth, his many sons, and all the ways the king had honored him and how he had elevated him above the other nobles and officials. "And that's not all," Haman added. "I'm the only person Queen Esther invited to accompany the king to the banquet she gave. And she has invited me along with the king tomorrow. But all this gives me no satisfaction as long as I see that Jew Mordecai sitting at the king's gate."
>
> His wife Zeresh and all his friends said to him, "Have a pole set up, reaching to a height of fifty cubits, and ask the king in the morning to have Mordecai impaled on it. Then go with the king to the banquet and enjoy yourself." This suggestion delighted Haman, and he had the pole set up.
>
> —Esther 5:9–14 NIV

BEAUTY TIP

Spending time thinking about what you have reduces the time to think about what you don't have.

MY FOUNDATION

MY FOUNDATION

A BEAUTIFUL SURRENDER

HAND IT OVER

The lady on the TV commercial walked briskly down the sidewalk, shopping bags hanging from her arms. She broke stride when she saw the stilettos in the shop window. She paused and lovingly looked at the bright red heels. Biting her nails, she lingered a bit longer. She started down the sidewalk again, trying to resist, but she didn't get past the door.

She tried on the shoes. Next scene, she is relaxing at home in front of the TV, popcorn bowl in her lap, feet propped up in red stilettos.

I know the feeling. It was tennis shoes for me. We were on a strict budget, but I tried on the way-cool tennis shoes marked twenty dollars over my limit anyway. They cushioned my feet in luxury and looked great from every angle. Even the kids would be impressed with these up-to-the-minute shoes. But twenty dollars over budget? I grudgingly put them back.

That isn't the end of the story.

I thought about the shoes all week. I wanted them—bad! The money barrier nagged until I wanted to rip up every budget document in the house. Those twenty stinking dollars irritated me. Why couldn't I let this go? It was just a pair of crazy shoes. I suddenly saw the truth: the reality that I couldn't afford the shoes had become greater than the fact that I didn't own them.

I prayed in anger over the stupid situation. "God, I'm tired of fighting against what I can't have. Please, please give me a spirit of contentment with what I can afford. I give up the shoes. Just help me be content." It was a small step, but it was the start of overcoming my angry emotions.

Emotional responses invade every part of our days, and these responses to troubles can determine whether we experience peace or remain caught in negative emotions. We need to be aware that our emotions powerfully affect our behavior. Choosing how we will respond ahead of time is the best beauty plan I can think of.

Since the shoe incident, I have adopted what I call *seize and surrender*. It's found in 2 Corinthians 10:5: **"We demolish arguments and every pretension that sets itself up against the knowledge of God, and we take captive every thought to make it obedient to Christ"** (NIV). I just love the mental picture of that verse. I imagine seizing a negative thought by its scrawny little neck and surrendering it to what Christ wants. So when thoughts come like, *I hate living on a strict budget* or *I look so fat in this dress* or *I'll never really do anything great for God,* I confess it to God, put the thought under his authority, and ask God to control my mind. This also works if I'm thinking something like, *My past is too colorful for God to forgive* or *That man's gonna pay for what he did to me.*

On the other hand, if I allow myself to dwell on those thoughts without intervention, I respond with feelings such as failure, anger, bitterness, hopelessness, or revenge.

I have come to the amazing revelation that God is big enough to handle our ugliness. And don't worry about admitting your nasty thoughts to God. As your mama always told you, he already knows.

Oh—the shoes? Several days later I returned to the store, contented to purchase a pair in my price range. As I approached the shoe display, a big red sticker caught my eye. It was on my shoes, and it read, "$20 off." Did God reward my surrender to his will? Maybe. But more importantly, I believe God was motivated by his glory. I was able to give God thanks and praise for the gift of his contentment. It just so happened that I received an extra blessing from it too.

And each time I put on my shoes, I can't help but remember the grace, goodness, and glory of my powerful Father as I surrender my mind to his ways.

The Esther Factor

King Xerxes responded in some emotionally charged circumstances. First, he reacted without much thought to Haman's request to kill the people he labeled disobedient. King Xerxes's course of action seems thoughtless and uncompassionate.

He then got angry and stormed out of the banquet hall when he found out he'd been deceived by Haman. However, he was determined to be fair and returned to administer swift justice to Haman for his lies. He admitted wrong had been done and subsequently gave Haman's wealth to Esther and Haman's position to Mordecai.

So even the king of Persia didn't always respond with grace and forethought. But it seems he recognized wrong priorities and decisions and was willing to correct them. We don't hear him say, "I'm sorry" or "I was wrong," but his actions indicate the king's change of heart and his desire to see that right prevailed. King Xerxes responded with compassion toward Esther and allowed the Jews to defend themselves when their enemies attacked.

Our human nature is going to trip us up and tempt us with negative emotions and actions. But we are wise if we realize our victory and peace rest in admitting our sin and seizing and surrendering our thoughts to God.

Did King Xerxes surrender his thoughts to God? We can't say directly from the text. But he granted every petition of Mordecai and Esther after the hanging of Haman. He couldn't help but see their devotion to a great and mighty God.

Our thoughts become our actions, and our actions are out there on display for the world. A thoughtful life surrendered to God, especially when problems abound, makes a powerful tool for the advance of the kingdom of God.

King Xerxes asked Queen Esther, "Who is he? Where is he—the man who has dared to do such a thing?"

Esther said, "An adversary and enemy! This vile Haman!"

Then Haman was terrified before the king and queen. The king got up in a rage, left his wine and went out into the palace garden. But Haman, realizing that the king had already decided his fate, stayed behind to beg Queen Esther for his life.

Just as the king returned from the palace garden to the banquet hall, Haman was falling on the couch where Esther was reclining.

The king exclaimed, "Will he even molest the queen while she is with me in the house?

As soon as the word left the king's mouth, they covered Haman's face.

Then Harbona, one of the eunuchs attending the king, said, "A pole reaching to a height of fifty cubits stands by Haman's house. He had it set up for Mordecai, who spoke up to help the king."

The king said, "Impale him on it!" So they impaled Haman on the pole he had set up for Mordecai. Then the king's fury subsided.

—Esther 7:5–10 NIV

BEAUTY TIP

Asking God for a spirit of contentment is step one in seize and surrender.

MY FOUNDATION

DAY
15

MY FOUNDATION

GOING FOR THE GOLD

THIS IS WORTH IT

This should be an interesting article, I thought. I began reviewing what the author had to say about some potential reactions to beauty products. But shortly into the article, I laughed so hard my mascara ran. The sentence read, "Most people can safely use most beauty products but sin reactions and other allergic problems are common."

It's so hard for a grade-school spelling champion not to notice misspelled words. And if we were to play Correct the Sentence, I know you'd say, "I'd like to buy a *K*, please," because I doubt the article intended to address our spiritual state.

But sin does react and cause us grief in many ways.

Let's just be honest. Sin is at the root of the problems in our lives. Whether the troubles come from this sinful world, from other people's decisions to wreak havoc, or from our own choices, they still hurt. We have pain. Seasons of trouble can be devastating. Problems can seem to weigh us down 24-7. And even if we are consciously surrendering our thought responses to God, it seems we spend twenty-four hours a day doing that too.

No doubt when we say "troubled man," we think of Job. Job experienced more in one season of testing than we will probably encounter in our entire lifetimes. Remember what happened to him? He lost his entire animal herd, every servant, all his sons and daughters, and to top that off his wife deserted her faith and nagged Job to curse God and die. Definitely more than a bad hair day.

At one point Job even felt like God had deserted him. "**If I go to the east, he is not there; if I go to the west, I do not find him. When he** is at work in the north, I do not see him; when he turns to the south, I catch no glimpse of him" (Job 23:8–9 NIV).

Ever felt like that? That God is nowhere to be found—except in other peoples' lives? I have. I recall one period of time when God seemed so far away, I entertained the thought, *Does God even exist?* And this was after being a Christian for more than thirty years.

Job's response to his problems surpasses beauty. He said, "**But he [God] knows the way that I take; when he has tested me, I will come forth as gold**" (Job 23:10 NIV).

Gold goes through an intense refining process to get to its state of holding diamonds. The gold in our favorite rings or necklaces experienced a high-intensity furnace to get out the impurities. And it's only through that process that gold can be considered pure.

The longer I try to be beautifully obedient, the more I realize there are some things we simply cannot accomplish, or know about God, until we go through the fire. It's during the fiery troubles that we see how big God is. We experience his faithfulness, and only then can we emerge more beautiful than when we went into the flames.

It may take a while. And you may have to do like I did. I had to choose to believe in the reality of God even when I didn't feel it. Even when I didn't experience him. It was a choice. Every. Single. Day.

But I think Job went a step further. He made a choice to endure through the fire and declared, when all was done, that he would be found fully devoted to God. What a beautiful declaration!

The Esther Factor

If Job's famous line is, "I will come forth as gold," then Esther's must be, "If I perish, I perish."

I'm thinking Esther's situation was a devastating season. Her issues were prompted by Haman's jealousy and prideful actions which caused Mordecai to make a request that left her shaking in her royal sandals. Talk about a sin reaction.

We don't know whether Esther ever despaired her situation to the point of doubting God's existence or felt so much pressure that she thought she couldn't go on. Maybe we are just supposed to know Esther experienced problems like us, concentrate on her obedience, and see how God can work miraculously when his children are faithful to him—no matter the intensity of the fire.

I doubt Esther's problems were made any easier just because she wore a crown and lived in a palace. What strikes me most when thinking about Esther is that she must have been a common person, just like me. So not only was she exposed to problems, like me, she also had the same potential feelings and emotions as any other red-blooded female. Her options were 1) do nothing to stop the murder edict, resulting in all her people getting slaughtered and possibly herself too when the king learned she was a Jew, or 2) go to the king to try and stop the edict and risk death to herself. I would want to know what's behind Door #3, wouldn't you? But Esther wasn't playing "Let's Make a Deal." Her choices were a matter of life and death.

Esther rose above the pit and emerged from the devastating plot with her royal crown of gold firmly intact. She considered the godly counsel of Mordecai that she quite possibly had been placed in the palace to save God's people from destruction. So Esther made a choice. Just like Job. Just like me. And just like anyone else who knows that trials will come, that they can refine us, and that we can come forth as gold.

One shining result of pitfalls is that they tend to magnify the power of God as he shows up to help us. Our problems give God a chance to work. It's through the fire that we come closer to God and become a greater witness of his power to the world.

> When Esther's words were reported to Mordecai, he sent back this answer: "Do not think that because you are in the king's house you alone of all the Jews will escape. For if you remain silent at this time, relief and deliverance for the Jews will arise from another place, but you and your father's family will perish. And who knows but that you have come to your royal position for such a time as this?"
>
> —Esther 4:12–14 NIV

BEAUTY TIP

Dealing with sin according to God's plan purifies us and glorifies God.

MY FOUNDATION

MY FOUNDATION

ESTHER LAUDER

THE REWARDS OF STAYING FAITHFUL

So, what do I do when I wake up tomorrow and I'm fifty?" I asked my husband, trying to hide my foreboding state of mind.

"Um . . . how about the same thing you did when you were forty-nine?"

Leave it to a man to be so practical—and on the eve of my half-century birthday. I needed some sympathy here. Or at the very least, fifty dollars so I could go to the spa.

Later that evening I tied on my exercise shoes, grabbed my weights, and hit the street. I had a few more hours to work on that forty-something body and needed to face the next half century looking as good as I could!

For two miles I envisioned what would happen when I woke up in the morning. Would I feel different? Would I look fifty? What does fifty feel like? Would I feel older? Maybe I just hoped I'd feel something. Would I remember my name? Then the most sobering thought of all: statistically speaking, my life was half over.

Well, I guess I could live to 101. My grandma's sisters lived that long . . .

My bizarre thoughts were interrupted by my neighbor as she rode by on her bike. "Hey, you're looking great, Karen."

Without breaking my stride, I hollered, "We'll see what tomorrow brings when I turn fifty. Thought I'd better walk today while I still can."

She laughed. "Well, you're doing the right thing!"

A lot of things can happen to our bodies as we experience more birthdays. But as the saying goes, having birthdays is better than the alternative. I started preparing for my fiftieth birthday when I turned forty-nine. My campaign was "50 by 50"—lose fifty pounds by the time I was fifty.

So I did what I do best: I thought about it for the next nine months. Then I panicked! But by the grace of God (and I mean that with every ounce of my then-forty-nine-year-old body), I began to make some changes.

I started on my major problem area—lack of exercise. I began walking. I walked in the July Kansas heat. I walked when I was tired. I busted out those tennis shoes even though it made me late getting to a meeting. (At least now I had an excuse for being late.)

Then I targeted the other biggie: food. I chose lean meat when I wanted a juicy quarter-pound cheeseburger. I ate fruit when chocolate called my name. I drank water when I heard the soda fizz through the refrigerator door.

Guess what? I didn't lose fifty pounds in those three remaining months; but I lost a reasonable amount of weight, inches disappeared, and I got to buy smaller pants.

So what happened when I turned fifty? I realized that when we are faithful and committed—even when we struggle and don't feel like it—with God's strength we will reap the rewards. There are rewards for staying faithful—in every area of life!

The Esther Factor

Of course there are much more eternal efforts in which to be faithful than weight loss. Being faithful to God's plan is the most important thing. But the wonderful thing about faithfulness is that God rewards it! **"And without faith it is impossible to please Him, for he who comes to God must believe that He is and that He is a rewarder of those who seek Him"** (Hebrews 11:6 NASB).

Esther shows us what being faithful to God looks like and the consequences of following him no matter the situation. Her actions reaped rewards, not only for herself but also for a whole race of people.

Let's put ourselves in Esther's sandals for a moment. While we're at it, let's try on her gown, crown, and jewelry. To start, we've already lived as a foreigner in a land with different customs than ours. We've been the exiles. When we were young, we experienced the death of our parents, and then we tried to maintain our composure as we were nominated for a beauty contest we never intended to enter.

Just when we got a handle on that, we found ourselves queen of this foreign land! Settling into palace life, we then heard our dear cousin Mordecai was in great distress. He sent us a message about a royal order to assassinate all of the Jewish people in the land. If that was not enough to drive us to a triple hot fudge sundae, Mordecai dropped the big one on us: go to the king and ask him to save us!

We knew the problems with that, however. Anyone who dared to enter the king's presence without being invited risked death unless the king held out his scepter as permission to enter. And it had been months since he'd asked for our company.

Well, how did those sandals feel? Ever have one of those years?

For Esther, this spanned the course of her young life and then a period of about five years once she reached the palace. Esther wore her sandals and the crown in a stately manner. She walked in beautiful obedience and faithfulness. She exposed Haman's deceitful plot, and the Jewish people's lives were spared.

The reward for Esther's faithfulness? She received all of Haman's wealth and estate, and Mordecai was given the scoundrel's position.

But Esther will receive her greatest reward when the rest of us faithful followers also get ours! The Bible says, **"I consider that our present sufferings are not worth comparing with the glory that will be revealed in us. . . . For our light and momentary troubles are achieving for us an eternal glory that far outweighs them all" (Romans 8:18; 2 Corinthians 4:17 NIV).**

The glory we will experience when we reach eternity will make all our earthly problems seem so trivial, I wonder if we'll even remember our struggles when we get to that side of heaven. So while we're here, our challenge is to keep focused on eternity and what is to come.

That same day King Xerxes gave Queen Esther the estate of Haman, the enemy of the Jews. And Mordecai came into the presence of the king, for Esther had told how he was related to her. The king took off his signet ring, which he had reclaimed from Haman, and presented it to Mordecai. And Esther appointed him over Haman's estate.

—Esther 8:1–2 NIV

BEAUTY TIP

Our troubles are so temporary. But the reward is coming, and it's eternal!

MY FOUNDATION

PART 3

THE POWER

Looking for Beauty in All the Wrong Places

EASY, NOT SMART

Beauty power is at my fingertips. Just a click on the keyboard and the Internet is glad to accommodate me with answers on any given beauty issue. The latest article I read promised I could "Look Younger by Monday."[3] This was Sunday, so I thought I'd see what overnight miracle awaited me. The article detailed several surefire methods to erase aging and possess refreshed skin by the time I returned to work on Monday.

Method #1: Puree blueberries for a mask to massage on the face.

Method #2: Mix honey, oatmeal, and few egg whites to form a paste. Apply to face and prop up your feet for ten minutes and bask in this oatmeal bath, after placing lukewarm green tea bags on the outside corners of each eye to reduce stress wrinkles.

Girl, I have to admit, I didn't try either of these. The mental pictures were much too bizarre. Are you with me here?

Suppose the kids ran in and saw me with pureed blueberries on my face. I figure they'd be wondering when the Smurfs got back into town. Or they'd think I had stopped breathing and call 9-1-1, and then I'd have to explain to paramedics why I had blueberries on my face.

Then I could picture myself with oatmeal packed on my face, feet up on the couch, relaxing with tea bags hanging off the sides of my face—and hubby walking in the door. After he realized it was actually me, I'm thinking he would wonder why his favorite breakfast was on my face.

Nope, I wasn't game to *face* either of those reactions!

We may be able to find all sorts of beauty solutions on the Internet; but where do we seek out solutions when we encounter problems trying to live God's plan? Plenty of voices vie for our attention, promising answers to our troubles. Sometimes our own selfish desires try to dictate our responses. Or maybe we turn to the myriad books and other media shouting messages of deliverance.

But God is the true source of power for his children. We talked at the start of our journey together about building on a foundation, and it's that foundation that provides the answers we need, especially when storms occur in our lives: "**Therefore everyone who** *hears these words of mine and puts them into practice* **is like a wise man who built his house on the rock. The rain came down, the streams rose, and the winds blew and beat against that house; yet it did not fall, because it had its foundation on the rock**" (Matthew 7:24–25 NIV, emphasis mine).

Rain really ruins a girl's foundation—but only the kind she wears on her face! A foundation on Jesus Christ helps us to withstand the rain and storms of life. As we listen to God and trust his ways, we can accomplish his plan for our lives.

THE ESTHER FACTOR

Talk about a storm that could test your foundation! This must have been it. When Queen Esther sent that message to find out what was ailing Mordecai, she had no idea the extent of the problem or what he was going to ask her to do. If Esther thought being an orphan in a foreign land or leaving Mordecai to go to the palace had been stressful, the request before her at this point must have registered at least a 7.2 on her stress scale.

However, remember what the beauty queen does? She didn't relieve the stress by buying a new outfit, getting a massage, or even basking in an oatmeal mask! She went before the Lord God Almighty, the foundation and power of her life.

How do we know it was God's power she sought? We've mentioned that neither God's name nor prayer is mentioned in the entire book of Esther. Yet even though those words, for some reason, were not penned in the book of Esther, their presence is seen by careful observation. Matthew Henry says in his commentary on Esther: "But, though the name of God is not in it, the finger of God is, directing many minute events for the bringing about of his people's deliverance."[4]

Esther could have chosen to listen to a variety of other counsel. She could have asked the opinion of her maids. Instead she requested them to fast with her. She could have looked to her own self for sheer determination and courage. That's what we're told today to do—look within!

But cousin Mordecai must have raised her right. Esther knew the most reliable source was not those around her, nor could she simply pull herself up by her own stiletto straps. She needed God!

We can be assured from Queen Esther's fasting and daring actions that this Jewish orphan knew the power of God—and that he was her source to turn to when life got tough.

When Mordecai learned of all that had been done, he tore his clothes, put on sackcloth and ashes, and went out into the city, wailing loudly and bitterly. But he went only as far as the king's gate, because no one clothed in sackcloth was allowed to enter it. In every province to which the edict and order of the king came, there was great mourning among the Jews, with fasting, weeping and wailing. Many lay in sackcloth and ashes.

When Esther's eunuchs and female attendants came and told her about Mordecai, she was in great distress. She sent clothes for him to put on instead of his sackcloth, but he would not accept them. Then Esther summoned Hathak, one of the king's eunuchs assigned to attend her, and ordered him to find out what was troubling Mordecai and why.

—Esther 4:1–5 NIV

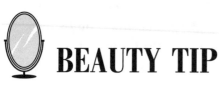

BEAUTY TIP

God gives the power to accomplish what he asks us to do.

MY FOUNDATION

MY FOUNDATION

POWER INCOGNITO

FEEL LIKE A ZERO?

I checked out at the doctor's office with a bit of trepidation. I had been experiencing considerable lower-back pain and chose to treat it with a round of chiropractic visits.

The first visit felt good, but I asked, "Should I feel any soreness from the treatment?"

"Drinking lots of water will help with any potential soreness," my chiropractor said. She handed me a cold bottle of water from her cooler and asked, "Do you drink a lot of water?"

"Does tea count?" I countered with a sheepish grin.

Her frown-that-was-supposed-to-look-like-a-smile told me it didn't. That's when she pulled out her "water is so good for you" sermon.

My burning question has always been, "What's the big deal about water anyway?" I've read the nutritional label: 0 calories, 0 carbohydrates, 0 protein, 0 vitamin A, 0 calcium, 0 vitamin C, 0 iron. Shouldn't that make it a bottle of nothing?

But everybody *and* the beauty industry proclaim the multibenefits of water. From skin and hair health to digestive health. From relieving headaches to losing weight. And from increased better moods to enhanced energy for your day.

Yet for some reason, I still don't care for water. With or without lemon, it's never my drink of choice. But I try to consume my share of the clear bottle of zero because of the reported health and beauty benefits. I'm attempting to convince myself it's my miracle power in disguise.

Even Jesus tried to market water. Actually, he was more on my side of the issue. He told an immoral woman at a water well that **"everyone who drinks this water will be thirsty again"** (John 4:13 niv). Maybe he didn't see the water benefit thing going on either, but apparently he had another water—living water—to offer this needy woman. Jesus went on to say, **"But whoever drinks the water I give him will never thirst. Indeed, the water I give him will become in him a spring of water welling up to eternal life"** (v. 14 NIV84).

The water Jesus offered is for eternal life—salvation. But this living water is also what gives us the power to live an abundant life after giving our hearts to God. Like we've said before, we weren't put here just to get saved and look cute! We have an abundant life waiting to be lived out, but we can't do it without the power of God.

Often this power doesn't come looking like we expect. It's not found in seminary training or a Christian conference experience. It does not come through our natural talents and abilities or by sheer determination to accomplish a task. God can use education, talents, and willingness, but the power is God himself working through us when we surrender everything to his authority and will. As we do this, God can work even through sinful, weak, seemingly zero people like us.

I often struggle, wondering how God could use a nobody like me. However, I've come to the conclusion that, although without God I'm nothing, with God I'm everything!

Isn't it amazing how God can take a zero and make it so useful? That's the power of God!

THE ESTHER FACTOR

I don't know about you, but blueberries, oatmeal, and water seem like some pretty unusual beauty options. And as mentioned before, an uneducated, inexperienced orphan like Esther might seem a rather unlikely nominee for saving a nation! But I wonder sometimes whether God purposely chooses a surprise option—an option that seems to rate a zero—to get his work done.

We see the amazing power of God working through many improbable people in the Bible. A little shepherd boy named David killed a terrorizing giant. A prostitute named Rahab helped the Israelite spies and saved her family when Jericho fell. Lowly, uneducated, outcast shepherds heard the first birth announcement of the Savior of the world.

That's not to mention some others who participated in getting God's work done but received only a one-line bio in the Bible:

"Here is a boy with five small barley loaves and two small fish" (John 6:9 NIV).

"As they [the disciples] were untying the colt, its owners asked, 'Why are you untying the colt?' They replied, 'The Lord needs it'" (Luke 19:33–34 NIV).

"As they were going out, they met a man from Cyrene, named Simon, and they forced him to carry the cross" (Matthew 27:32 NIV).

These people might not have seemed like much. They were just faces among the crowd, maybe zeroes in the eyes of the world. Yet God used them to get his mission accomplished and his power revealed. I wonder sometimes whether God even considers our abilities, talents, or credentials when he wants to really display his power. After all, he seems to find the most unqualified person in the world's eyes to get work done. Maybe he does that so people will have to acknowledge the power is God's power, not human ability.

Esther certainly is among those who inspire us to think outside the box about God's power. She stepped out in beautiful obedience, and God's power was ignited.

On the third day Esther put on her royal robes and stood in the inner court of the palace, in front of the king's hall. The king was sitting on his royal throne in the hall, facing the entrance. When he saw Queen Esther standing in the court, he was pleased with her and held out to her the gold scepter that was in his hand. So Esther approached and touched the tip of the scepter.

Then the king asked, "What is it, Queen Esther? What is your request? Even up to half the kingdom, it will be given you."

"If it pleases the king," replied Esther, "let the king, together with Haman, come today to a banquet I have prepared for him."

—Esther 5:1–4 NIV

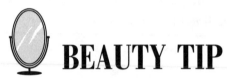 **BEAUTY TIP**

Think outside the box and see what God's power does through you.

MY FOUNDATION

MY FOUNDATION

3-IN-1 LIPSTICK

MORE THAN YOUR AVERAGE LIP SERVICE

I enviously eyed the magazine model's sleek, slender thighs. Could I ever have thighs like that? Apparently all I had to do was buy her brand of skin-firming lotion to end up with picture-perfect legs. I jotted down the name of the product and snatched some up on my next shopping trip. My secret desire? Eliminate cellulite and make my legs as thin as hers. Oh, a girl can dream!

An ad for a three-in-one lipstick promised more grandiose results: line your lips, fill them in , and plump them up as a finale. The Big and Healthy 3-in-1.

Is it just me or are you also skeptical of products that can do it all? I try to stay away from any beauty product that promises to plump anything. My body parts have been doing a fine job of plumping themselves for years now, thank you very much. But I always wonder whether these miracle products are all they're advertised to be.

Or are they just giving me lip service?

When I was young, my dad referred to people who were all talk and no action as simply giving him lip service. He might have been talking about me.

Our lips are used for an important purpose when we are following God—and it doesn't matter if they're filled or plumped. Using our lips in prayer releases God's power. Prayer is the key to experiencing obedience to God's will. We could write a whole book just on prayer, but that's already been done by some very competent people. So let's just go over a few prayer basics.

Jesus told us to pray. He told us to ask, seek, and knock. He instructed his followers how to pray. He went away and prayed by

himself, as well as with his disciples. We're simply doing what Jesus
commanded and modeled. Charles Surgeon, famed nineteenth-century
pastor and author, said, "Whether we like it or not, asking is the rule of
the kingdom."

We don't have because we don't ask (James 4:2). Sometimes when I
realize I'm not experiencing God's strength, I have to ask myself what part
of that verse I don't understand. And there is nothing too small for us to
ask God to consider.

Prayer takes persistence. While exercising at my favorite gym, I
overheard an employee's phone conversation with a disgruntled customer.
The employee hung up and said, "She wants to cancel her membership,
and she's only been here twice." Twice wasn't going to cut it for exercise.
And sometimes twice isn't enough in prayer. That's why Luke recorded,
**"Then Jesus told his disciples a parable to show them that they
should always pray and not give up"** (Luke 18:1 NIV).

There must have been an important reason why Jesus taught so
much on prayer. Did he want to make sure we thoroughly understood its
necessity? Sometimes we don't understand why a prayer doesn't seem to
be answered or why it's taking so long. But our job is to give prayer *proper*
lip service—pray, pray, and then pray some more. Prayer isn't something
to check off our spiritual to-do lists; it's the key to the power of the true
beauty of obedience. As we come to God in confession and humility, God
will give us the power for what he wants us to do.

The Esther Factor

OK, by now we all realize the word *prayer* isn't in the book of Esther. But we've noted that Esther's fasting indicates a prayer life. So what's up with fasting? What did Esther hope to accomplish with it?

Fasting in the Old Testament is often associated with distress or some potential impending doom or destruction. Israel and the prophet Samuel fasted in repentance before they went up to fight against the Philistines (1 Samuel 7). Daniel fasted and prayed in response to learning of the seventy years of desolation for Israel (Daniel 9:1–3). The prophet Nehemiah fasted and prayed over the destruction of Jerusalem and its walls (Nehemiah 1:3–4).

"Fast"-forward to New Testament days. We see Jesus himself fasted for forty days (Matthew 4). He later refereed arguments about the issue. Apparently certain religious people were drawing attention to themselves and their piety. He straightened out everyone's motives for fasting when he said that no one should be able to tell by your appearance that you are fasting (Matthew 6:16–18). Matthew 9:14 records that John the Baptist's followers came to Jesus and just happened to mention that they and the religious leaders fasted, and why didn't his followers do the same?

So fasting was not uncommon in biblical times. And Esther used the practice for a specific purpose—to earnestly seek God in a difficult situation.

The late Bill Bright, American evangelist and founder of Campus Crusade for Christ, gave this added dimension for us in this century: "Fasting and prayer can restore the loss of the 'first love' for your Lord and result in a more intimate relationship with Christ." [5]

Do you need restoration with your heavenly Father? Have the problems of life come between you and God? Have struggles overwhelmed you to the point of depression? Do you earnestly need intervention from the one who has power to overcome? Maybe God is calling you to fast as you continue to pray. Information abounds on the subject. Some research and careful consideration may be the springboard to releasing God's power in your life.

Esther simply fasted and prayed as an obedient seeker of God's power, and power is what she experienced.

> Then Esther sent this reply to Mordecai: "Go, gather together all the Jews who are in Susa, and fast for me. Do not eat or drink for three days, night or day. I and my attendants will fast as you do. When this is done, I will go to the king, even though it is against the law. And if I perish, I perish." So Mordecai went away and carried out all of Esther's instructions.
>
> —Esther 4:15–17 NIV

BEAUTY TIP

Research the topic of fasting and prayerfully consider whether God is calling you to fast.

MY FOUNDATION

MY FOUNDATION

KNOW A GOOD HAIRAPIST?

GETTIN' A LITTLE HELP FROM MY FRIENDS

Hi, my name is Karen, and I have HOCD—hair obsessive-compulsive disorder. OK, it's out in the open. I've done step one. To recover from any addiction, isn't step one always admitting you have a problem? So there you have it—I have this bizarre obsession with my hair.

This won't surprise those closest to me. Well, except my husband. He seldom notices, even when I've had my twelfth haircut in three months.

"What do you think of my hair?" I'll ask. He eyes me cautiously, squints, and bites his lip. He's probably wondering whether this is a trick question. I imagine the conversation in his mind: *Did she get it cut? Is she letting it grow? Another color possibly? Did she part it on the other side? Is she contemplating a new style? Trying out a different shampoo? What does she want me to say?*

Oh, and he is as smooth as he is honest. He finally replies, "You look lovely in any hairstyle, dear."

Step two in my hair-recovery program is sticking close to my *hairapist*. You know what a hairapist is, don't you? A hairapist is someone to whom you trust the very hairs on your head. My hairapist understands that a bad-hair day ranks right up there with a national disaster and a good-hair day is grounds for throwing a party the size of Mardi Gras. She also knows the number of gray hairs on my head yet agrees my hair is whatever color I say it is!

But she's more than a dresser of hair. When I slip into her magic chair, she asks, "How's it going?" Then her ears and heart work just as hard as her hands. While she snips my tresses, she listens to and responds to the other hairy situations in my life. She reminds me I can't lock up my teens until they're thirty, that sometimes I need to control my control freakiness, and that I am a redeemed daughter of God even when I think I've failed miserably. And the best part—when it's time to pay, she charges only for the haircut, not the therapy and rehab.

Sometimes God works his power through the friends he gives us. And we all need a little help from our friends, don't we? Our girlfriends can help us when the going gets tough. They can remind us that God loves, forgives, and gives us grace for whatever we've done, and sometimes we just need them to push us back into this thing called life.

I have often spent hours sitting and talking with my girlfriends. We've even closed down a few restaurants in our time. When hubby is amazed that all we did was talk, I remind him, "You should be glad you didn't have to listen to me for three hours."

We women need each other. And one would think it was a woman who wrote this, but King Solomon paralleled the wisdom of a woman when he wrote, **"Two are better than one, because they have a good return for their work: If one falls down, his friend can help him up. But pity the man who falls and has no one to help him up!"** (Ecclesiastes 4:9–10 NIV).

THE ESTHER FACTOR

OK, the Bible doesn't call them girlfriends, but they must have had some of the key ingredients we need in our circles of friends. Esther's maids, as the Bible calls them, were close to her. They probably knew about the day-to-day affairs of their queen. Maybe it was even their job to shuffle through the closets of royal fashion wear to select Esther's daily attire. I can picture them swooping Esther's hair into the latest updo and precisely applying just the right makeup.

And apparently Esther was intimate enough with her maids that she felt she could ask them to go through her difficult situation with her. She asked them to fast with her.

Esther was willing to bear her distress with her maids. Are you as vulnerable with your friends? Are you willing to expose your deepest problems, even sins, to them? Girls, our friends can't help us if we act as if we're an impenetrable fortress of strength, that nothing ever hurts or affects us. We've got to let our friends inside.

Esther's maids must have loved her—they were willing to give up three days of food! Ouch! I have to admit, I like to play it a little safer than that. I'll pray for my friends—but give up nine meals and some snacks? Am I that good a friend?

Chances are, most of the time, our friends ask a lot less of us than that. Our sacrifices come more in the way of time and energy. It takes endurance and emotional support to help our girlfriends through the storms of life. Are we willing to be that friend someone needs?

Oh, the power that comes when friends unite! After Esther and her maids fasted for three days, Esther readied herself and went to King Xerxes. And prayers were answered. The king admitted her to the throne room, and negotiations began. Not only that, the end of the story is just as miraculous.

God's power was at work. And his power continues to work today when we join with each other and seek him. Maybe that's why James 5:16 says, **"Therefore confess your sins to each other and pray for each other so that you may be healed. The prayer of a righteous man [and woman!] is powerful and effective"** (NIV84).

Maybe you're thinking, *But, Karen, I don't have any friends.* First, if your foundation is God, he is the very best friend. He's with you always. Next, God knows the importance of friends, so ask him to send you a friend to encourage you and one you can encourage in return. Then keep a watch and see how God answers your prayer.

King Xerxes replied to Queen Esther and to Mordecai the Jew, "Because Haman attacked the Jews, I have given his estate to Esther, and they have impaled him on the pole he set up. Now write another decree in the king's name in behalf of the Jews as seems best to you, and seal it with the king's signet ring—for no document written in the king's name and sealed with his ring can be revoked."

At once the royal secretaries were summoned—on the twenty-third day of the third month, the month of Sivan. They wrote out all Mordecai's orders to the Jews, and to the satraps, governors and nobles of the 127 provinces stretching from India to Cush. These orders were written in the script of each province and the language of each people and also to the Jews in their own script and language. Mordecai wrote in the name of King Xerxes, sealed the dispatches with the king's signet ring, and sent them by mounted couriers, who rode fast horses especially bred for the king.

The king's edict granted the Jews in every city the right to assemble and protect themselves; to destroy, kill and annihilate the armed men of any nationality or province who might attack them and their women and children, and to plunder the property of their enemies.

—Esther 8:7–11 NIV

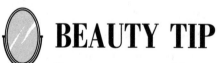

BEAUTY TIP

Be transparent and let your girlfriends help you.

MY FOUNDATION

MY FOUNDATION

LADIES IN WAITING

BEAUTY IN HIS TIME

Hairapists are great, huh? When I leave my stylist, the miraculous power that's been worked on my hair leaves me on cloud nine. But something drastic happens by the next morning. I get up excited to fix that new 'do, wash my hair quickly, and start the styling process. And for me, it is a process. I'm what you'd call hair challenged. I might be HOCD, but the energies that go into my obsessiveness falter when it comes to actually fixing the hair. I just can't seem to get it right, especially after a new cut.

Someone once explained to me that hair is "shocked" when it gets cut. And I actually read an Internet discussion on the bizarre topic of shocked hair. Amazing! Opinions varied, but the shock story was a popular belief.

Shocked or not, my hair definitely has a mind of its own after a cut. It refuses to cooperate. So I wait. And wait. And wait. Then after repeated stylings over the next few days, one morning I shout, "Hallelujah!" I'm back on cloud nine with the hair, and life is good.

I'd like to avoid getting my hair cut at all. However, even those who grow long hair still get their hair trimmed to eliminate split ends. The professionals say it promotes healthy hair. But waiting for it to grow back out—or in my case, into manageable strands—is as enjoyable as waiting on hold for Internet customer service. It takes forever and keeps me wondering what exactly is going on at the other end.

Ever feel like that with God? We know he's promised to come through for us, be there for us, and answer our prayers. We believe he wants to give us the power to help us work through our problems. But there we are, with our brand-new hairstyles, smack in the middle of a situation that seems to be going nowhere, waiting. And waiting. And waiting. Ever wonder what God is doing when you're in that waiting room?

I'm not sure the question should be, What is God doing? but What are we doing? If we find ourselves in the waiting room, maybe we need to look to see if we're doing all we should be. Are you beautifully obedient in the other areas of your life, or do you need to confess some old junk? Do you continually praise God in spite of your circumstances, or do you need some thought transplants? Can you acknowledge God is still in control, or do you tend to bail out on waiting for God's response and take matters into your own hands?

There are a lot of temptations in the waiting room: discouragement, bitterness, anger, and negativity, to name a few. But they lead nowhere. Instead, Isaiah 40:31 clues us in that **"those who wait on the Lord shall renew their strength"** (NIV). What does "wait" mean here? Other translations use *hope* and *trust*.

Wait, hope, and trust—our buddies in the waiting room! We wait because sometimes God's plans just take time. We hope because God has rescued us before. And we trust because God is God—and he is powerfully faithful!

The Esther Factor

Details, details. I sure would like more particulars than God gives in some of the narratives in the Bible. Of course, being a spiritually mature child of God (and extremely humble), I assume God has reasons for giving us exactly the information he did. However, that doesn't keep me from wondering about the missing details.

Take, for instance, the three days Esther and her maids spent fasting and waiting. There is one line about this. Uno. Mordecai has asked Esther to visit the king and expose Haman's evil intentions to kill the Jews, so she decides to fast for three days. But my inquiring mind wants to know what Esther was doing while she waited. Did she almost back out? Compose a contingency plan? Did she fire any questions to her God about his existence? Did she feel alone? Were there sleepless nights? Did she ever get angry, even though she knew she needed to do the job?

What we do know is that she was content to fast for three days. I know what you're thinking: *If only I had to wait for three measly days, I'd be content too!* I've felt like that. One season of my life was spent waiting for a child to come back to God. I got to the point in the waiting room where I thought, *I could handle the rebellion, God, if you'd just let me know when all this is going to end.* Guess what? God didn't give me a time line. I just had to wait, hope, and trust.

If you think Esther had it easy with only three days of waiting, think again. After those three days, she still had to approach the king, be allowed into his presence, and expose Haman and his evil scheme.

But the king couldn't just cancel his edict. Royal decrees could not be cancelled. However, Mordecai was allowed to issue an order in the king's name to override the first murder decree. This decree allowed the Jews to defend themselves against Haman's armies.

Then Esther entered the next waiting room. She spent the next eight months waiting to see whether the Jews could prevail over their enemies when they attacked. She must have waited with hope and trust because she had certainly seen the power of God's hand in the previous months. And remembering the faithfulness of God is a joyous and productive thing to do in the waiting room.

> Esther again pleaded with the king, falling at his feet and weeping. She begged him to put an end to the evil plan of Haman the Agagite, which he had devised against the Jews. Then the king extended the gold scepter to Esther and she arose and stood before him.
>
> "If it pleases the king," she said, "and if he regards me with favor and thinks it the right thing to do, and if he is pleased with me, let an order be written overruling the dispatches that Haman son of Hammedatha, the Agagite, devised and wrote to destroy the Jews in all the king's provinces. For how can I bear to see disaster fall on my people? How can I bear to see the destruction of my family?"
>
> —Esther 8:3–6 NIV

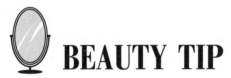

BEAUTY TIP

Exercise your hope, trust, and thankfulness in the waiting room.

MY FOUNDATION

_____

_____

_____

_____

_____

_____

_____

_____

_____

_____

_____

_____

_____

_____

_____

_____

_____

_____

_____

_____

_____

MY FOUNDATION

THE POWER OF BIG

MORE THAN YOU CAN IMAGINE

A survey asked men, "What scares you about women?" The answers were rather amusing. One man said, "Too much makeup. I've always been weirded out by mimes and clowns, so it may be related."

Hmm, ladies wearing much makeup, take note.

An important executive said what scared him about women is "their power. Women have all the power when it comes to men, because with a bat of their lashes, a look, a sweetness in their voice, women can get men to do anything. It's almost a superhuman feat, and that's petrifying."[6]

Hmm, ladies working for executives, take note.

This man may be right about how women sway men, but I'm not so sure I'd call that legitimate power. Sounds a bit more like persuasion than power. But what do I know? I'm probably just a woman who wears too much make up, bats my eyes, and tries to use my superhuman feats to get my husband to take me out to eat instead of watching *Monday Night Football*.

There is, however, a power that is genuine, miraculous, and downright huge. It's the power that created the world with a simple word. It's the power that caused women past child-bearing age and a virgin to have children. It's the power that turned a murderer into an apostle passionate for the cause of Christ. It held back seas and kept the sun from shining, and it caused pagan kings to acknowledge the one true living God.

God's power is *big*. I don't know about you, but I have a hard time wrapping my pretty little brain around the immenseness of God. It's unfathomable, way out of my realm of understanding. However, the apostle Paul said, "**I want to know Christ and the power of his resurrection**" (Philippians 3:10 NIV84). Talk about a man who could have believed he had near-superhuman power. Paul could have boasted that he started following the law at eight days old when he was circumcised, that he was of Benjamin's tribe and the best Jew of all Jews—faultlessly, legalistically righteous, and zealous against the church. (Try to put that on a resume and see if anyone believes you.)

Yet it was simply rubbish to him. What he wanted to experience was the power that raised Jesus Christ from the grave. And that is big power!

But sometimes we turn big into a problem. We think God's power is so big, it's out of our experiential realm. It's for super saints, missionaries, and our godly grandmas. Yes, God's power is huge, but God made it as tangible and personal as he could by coming to earth wrapped in the skin of Jesus. Then he died on the cross to make sure we had a way to experience the powerful, abundant life.

Most of us can accept the fact that Jesus died for us, so why can't we accept that his power is also available in us to finish the purpose for which he made us?

This life-giving power will transcend any problem we ever encounter as we follow God. In fact, no problem will ever be greater than God's power to overcome it. And he chooses to display his power through us and to us. His power gives us strength when we are tired of the whole ordeal. His power gives us wisdom when we think we've exhausted all possible options. And his power sometimes just holds us when all we can do is cry.

There is no other person, philosophy, or plan that brings strength as well as peace. Reach out and grab big and let God work through you!

THE ESTHER FACTOR

Esther lived in preresurrection years. However, she must have heard Jewish history through the years at the side of her cousin Mordecai. Hearing stories of how God worked in the lives of Abraham, Isaac, and Jacob couldn't help but strengthen her trust when she needed God the most.

I can't prove it, but I'm willing to use my superhuman strength here and convince you that Esther heard that her great-grandfather twenty times removed, named Abraham, had a baby when he was about a century old. And how that baby, named Isaac (her grandfather nineteen times removed), was about to be sacrificed on an altar when God miraculously provided a ram in the bushes as a substitute.

I bet she heard about another member of her family tree who wrestled with God and how God changed that relative's name from Jacob to Israel. And how could she forget about her ancestors who lived in bondage in Egypt and then walked on dry land through the Red Sea to escape that slavery? I know she must have heard about them wandering for forty years in a desert, their sandals not wearing out and supper falling from the heavens.

I'm thinking Esther perused the family scrapbook and saw how her Jewish relatives conquered Jericho and many other cities on their way to the Promised Land. And how time and again when her people disobeyed God, they later returned to him because they had seen Jehovah's faithfulness and miraculous powers throughout their history.

Esther must have been thoroughly familiar with God's working through the lives of those who had gone on before her. What courage that must have given her to rise up and and be used to save, once again, God's chosen people.

The power that Esther had always heard about and the power she experienced is the same power available to us today. In fact, we have a New Testament Scripture that gives us confidence to follow that same powerful God: **"Now to him who is able to do immeasurably more than all we ask or imagine, according to his power, that is at work within us"** (Ephesians 3:20 NIV).

We don't even have to bat our eyes. We just come before God with humble, trusting spirits and see what his supernatural power can do through us.

> When Mordecai left the king's presence, he was wearing
> royal garments of blue and white, a large crown of gold
> and a purple robe of fine linen. And the city of Susa held a
> joyous celebration. For the Jews it was a time of happiness
> and joy, gladness and honor. In every province and in
> every city to which the edict of the king came,
> there was joy and gladness among the Jews, with feasting
> and celebrating. And many people of other nationalities
> became Jews because fear of the Jews had seized them.
>
> —Esther 8:15–17 NIV

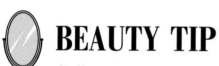

BEAUTY TIP

God's power is huge, but it can live inside of you through his Spirit.

MY FOUNDATION

MY FOUNDATION

TRUST HIM ON THIS

HE'S GOT IT COVERED

I'm beginning to think I'm an "articleaholic." If I see a great title, I can't resist reading what follows, even if I should be doing something important like plucking my eyebrows or changing my toenail polish. A recent article titled "What Men Don't Know about Women" was no exception. I mean, what female wouldn't want to read that? However, after reflecting on the article, I think I would have titled it "Guys, Trust Us Women on This One."

There were great nuggets of truth in the article, but my version of the article would have included info like, "Trust us on this one, men—we women are naturally self-conscious. It's not by choice. It's a genderwide condition." Another insight would be, "Trust us on this one, men—we women really do want dessert. We just want you to order it." And indulge me with just one more. "Trust us, men—when we ask which outfit we should wear, you can pretty much count on us going with the one you didn't choose. Yes, we asked your opinion, but that was just a stalling technique and to appear that we were getting some outside advice."

If only we could get the guys to trust us on this woman stuff. They would sail along in our relationships better if they just accepted those facts and others like these:

We won't always make sense to you, but it's perfectly logical in our minds.

We want you to be strong, but we want our own way.

We don't want a minute-by-minute replay of the football game, but you'd better remember every detail when our friend calls about the birth of her newborn.

When you tell us we're beautiful, expect us to act like we have no idea what you're talking about, but keep telling us.

When we ask if you like our hair, trust us—there is something different about our hair! You may not think so, but your safest answer is, "I absolutely love it like that."

Men, just trust us.

Maybe we women need a reminder of the importance of trust too. There are probably myriad of male perspectives we'd be better off simply trusting instead of trying to understand.

But when it comes to trusting in God and his power, sometimes our trust wanes. We question the path God seems to be leading. We think our plans might work better.

I saw this in 3-D when our family went on a trip to a city we had visited before. Our destination in that city was new to us, however, so we printed directions off the Internet. Reading over the map before we departed, we thought that at a certain juncture we would turn right, but the printed directions told us to turn left. We knew we'd have to check out that turn carefully.

When we got close to the area in question, we saw detour signs. Fortunately the diversion was only a looped detour ramp. But it was enough of a loop that it caused us to turn left at the top of the ramp, just as the directions had specified. This put us back on the road where we would have turned right without the detour. We got a lesson in trusting the power of a source outside of our limited knowledge.

It requires that kind of trust to follow God. But when we do, we experience his power. The truth is that we will never come to know God fully in his power until we come to trust fully in his providence. Often we think we know the way; we can't, however, know what's ahead or if God is going to take us on a detour to get us better prepared for the rest of the trip. In the end, we will get to our destination if we just trust and obey his leadership.

In his providential care, God has blazed a path for our lives. As we trust him, we will stay on the safety and peace of that path. We need to believe that he knows the right way—even on the detours.

THE ESTHER FACTOR

Mordecai and Esther had many chances to exercise their faith and trust. Mordecai blew the whistle on two murder schemes—one to kill King Xerxes and another to kill the Jewish people in the king's province of Susa. He probably realized this could have backfired, causing the plotters to seek revenge, but he was willing to take that risk. I'm convinced he had confidence in something bigger than himself.

Esther, too, probably thought trust in God was all she had. She was living in a palace in a non-Jewish country, and I doubt she had a weekly women's Bible study group to support her. Yes, she had her maids to fast with her when the heat really turned up, but that small group of women still turned their faith and attention to their source of power, God.

Just because Esther and Mordecai exercised their faith didn't mean it was easy. So how did they "just have faith"? I'm going to use my superhuman strength here again to submit that maybe, just maybe, family history had repeated the story of their forefather Abram, who **"believed the Lord, and he credited it to him as righteousness" (Genesis 15:6** NIV**).**

The context of that verse comes right after Abram questions God about his childlessness. God had promised him years ago he would have many descendants. I wonder if Abram felt like he was on a v-e-r-y long detour. So when he questioned God, God told Abram to look up and count the stars—and his family would be that abundant. I'm not sure whether Abram attempted to actually count those stars, but he understood God was making a promise to him—and he simply chose to believe it.

So how did Esther and her cousin "just have faith"? If indeed they heard about God's promises coming to pass in their Jewish history, they simply chose to sink their roots in that faithful God.

We can make the same choice. God's Word is full of his faithfulness. Will you continue to believe and trust in God as your source of power for living? If you do, I know God will keep every last one of his promises to be with you and strengthen you. And if I can invoke superhuman strength one last time, I'd like to shout, "Trust me on this one!"

On the thirteenth day of the twelfth month, the month of Adar, the edict commanded by the king was to be carried out. On this day the enemies of the Jews had hoped to overpower them, but now the tables were turned and the Jews got the upper hand over those who hated them. The Jews assembled in their cities in all the provinces of King Xerxes to attack those determined to destroy them. No one could stand against them, because the people of all the other nationalities were afraid of them. And all the nobles of the provinces, the satraps, the governors and the king's administrators helped the Jews, because fear of Mordecai had seized them. Mordecai was prominent in the palace; his reputation spread throughout the provinces, and he became more and more powerful.

The Jews struck down all their enemies with the sword, killing and destroying them, and they did what they pleased to those who hated them.

—Esther 9:1–5 NIV

BEAUTY TIP

We come to trust fully in God as we trust fully in his plan for our lives.

MY FOUNDATION

MY FOUNDATION

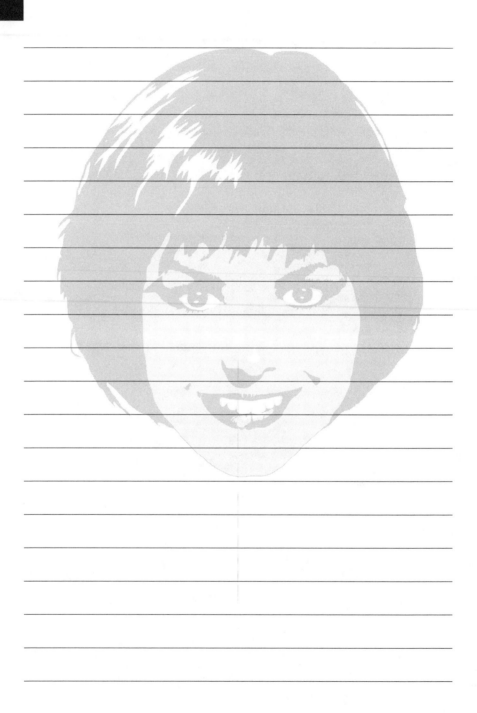

DRESS FOR SUCCESS

GOD'S WARDROBE

I hit the summer clearance racks for our upcoming trip to Australia. It was fall in the States, so it was spring down under, and that made for great timing on the leftover summer merchandise. It didn't take long to find a perfect $4.99 buy of the season—fabulous lime green capris. OK—maybe you wouldn't put *fabulous* and *lime green* in the same sentence, but did you catch that price?

My children have warned me before about my clothing choices and colors, so I thought I'd model the capris and get some input. I pranced on my imaginary living room runway and targeted my husband first, knowing he'd be proud of the price. "They were only $4.99! I know the color is a bit bright, but would you be embarrassed to be seen with me in Australia in these pants?"

Maybe I was just asking for it with a question like that, but he cautiously answered, "Would *you* want to be seen in Australia in those pants?"

I wasn't giving up. The teen was next. He covered his eyes, as if the lime green blinded him, and begged, "No, no, no," and ran out of the room, mumbling something about never wearing them in public when I was with him.

Did I take those lime green capris to Australia? You bet I did, and I have the pictures to prove it.

I'll admit I can be fashion challenged in the physical world, but there is another world I'm more concerned about. There is a heavenly wardrobe God wants his children to wear. It's not much of a fashion statement, but apparently it's effective in the spiritual realm. In fact, it gives us power for living. The apostle Paul calls it the "armor of God."

Armor may not have been on your fashion radar screen, but let's take a quick look at it. The exact dressing instructions are found in **Ephesians 6:10–17**; however, here is a crash course on our spiritual wardrobe:

Belt of truth. Obeying God means in everything. We need to be truth tellers and truth thinkers to experience God's power. God doesn't mix with half-truths, lies, and deception. **"The Lord hates . . . a lying tongue"** (**Proverbs 6:16–17** NIV).

Breastplate of righteousness. We are gifted with righteousness when we give our hearts to God. This gift helps us choose right, think right, and do right. It empowers us just knowing we are **"created to be like God in true righteousness and holiness"** (**Ephesians 4:24** NIV).

Shoes of the gospel of peace. God's power is shown when his children spread his gospel and walk in peace. We must be at peace ourselves. We can't give away what we don't have. **"How beautiful on the mountains are the feet of those who bring good news, who proclaim peace"** (**Isaiah 52:7** NIV).

Shield of faith. Satan will try to shoot arrows of doubt and fear at us. Our faith and trust in God leaves Satan shaking in his boots. Faith (our determined belief) is God's power used against the enemy. **"This is the victory that has overcome the world, even our faith"** (**1 John 5:4** NIV).

Helmet of salvation. Our salvation brings us peace of mind. Protect your mind and remind yourself often of your salvation and the power it affords you. **"I am not ashamed of the gospel, because it is the power of God for the salvation of everyone who believes"** (**Romans 1:16** NIV).

Sword of the Spirit. This is our power manual—the Bible. It is truth for confusion, wisdom for decisions, and comfort for discouragement. **"For the Word of God is living and active. Sharper than any double-edged sword . . ."** (**Hebrews 4:12** NIV).

The wardrobe of God. Put it on every morning, and you can be clothed with God's power.

The Esther Factor

I wonder how many royal gowns a queen of Persia would own. King Xerxes was quite wealthy. During his first recorded banquet in the book of Esther, he displayed all his wealth for 180 days! So I would hope his First Lady had a well-stocked wardrobe. I bet she didn't have to shop the clearance racks.

Even though she didn't know about the apostle Paul's spiritual-wardrobe description, we can compare Queen Esther's actions with this heavenly attire:

Belt of truth. Telling the truth is what posed the greatest risk to Esther. She launched the most dangerous event of her life with a challenge to expose deceit and lies. Being a truth teller is risky business, but God empowers us with boldness when we choose to do so. Esther certainly passes the truth test.

Breastplate of righteousness. If indeed stories of righteous decisions and actions were passed down through the generations, Esther also exemplifies having a solid breastplate. Her decisions to do the right thing must have empowered and encouraged her as she continued to see God work. There's nothing like the power of God working through us to embolden us to do the right thing again the next time.

Shoes of the gospel of peace. Esther's exposure of Haman's deceitful plot led to peace for the Jews and others in the land. Even though the Jews were allowed to defend against, and even kill, the armies that attacked them, God's peace came when right prevailed. After God's justice was satisfied with the elimination of these enemies, many in the land became Jews. When word of the one true God is spread and embraced, peace reigns.

Shield of faith. Yesterday we talked about the faith of Esther. Living in bold faith is a powerful deflector of Satan's agenda. He simply cannot get his way when we live a life that says, "I believe my God. He's big. He's bold. He promised, and he will come through for me."

Helmet of salvation. If you want a deep theological answer to, "How were people saved before Jesus came to this earth and died?"

seek out your pastor or a trusted Bible teacher. We do know that salvation comes through a relationship with God. Esther knew her God. Her relationship not only afforded her the salvation of God's grace and mercy, but it was his power that brought physical salvation to the endangered Jewish people living in Persia.

Sword of the Spirit. Ephesians 6:17 says, "Take . . . the sword of the Spirit, which is the word of God." We are so accustomed to the phrasing "the word of God" to mean the printed Bible as we know it in our day. But the "word of God" for Esther may more likely have been literal—the actual words of God. Esther used the sword of the Spirit as she experienced God moving in her heart and life, which enabled her to act courageously.

It doesn't matter what era we live in. When we dress in God's power, we can expect God will give us courage for whatever he asks us to do.

> So the king and Haman went to Queen Esther's banquet, and as they were drinking wine on the second day, the king again asked, "Queen Esther, what is your petition? It will be given you. What is your request? Even up to half the kingdom, it will be granted."
>
> Then Queen Esther answered, "If I have found favor with you, Your Majesty, and if it pleases you, grant me my life—this is my petition. And spare my people—this is my request. For I and my people have been sold to be destroyed, killed and annihilated. If we had merely been sold as male and female slaves, I would have kept quiet, because no such distress would justify disturbing the king."
>
> —Esther 7:1–4 NIV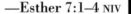

BEAUTY TIP

God's heavenly wardrobe—don't leave home without it.

MY FOUNDATION

PART 4

THE NEW YOU

APPLYING THE FOUNDATION

LEAVING THE UGLY

FORGETTING, FORGIVING, AND FORGING

That memorable Sunday years ago, as I greeted people after church, one of the congregation's most proper women came and shook my hand.

"How are you today?" I asked, shaking her thin, aging hand.

"I'm fine," she replied. Then she touched my shoulder ever so lightly and added, "I think you're gaining a little weight, aren't you?"

You know the Bible verse that says, "**Set a guard over my mouth, O Lord**" (Psalm 141:3 NKJV)? I'm living proof that we can pray a verse some months before and God actually remembers it. Because that is the only reason I didn't say what popped into my not-so-lovely brain.

My first thought was, *Oh, thank you. I was afraid nobody would notice.* That was followed by, *I've worked real hard at this. You just made my day.* But God is good, and he guarded my mouth.

Several months after that, I encountered a woman I hadn't seen in a while. I smiled and said, "Hi, Mary. It's been a long time since I've seen you."

She quizzically looked at me, thought for a moment, and said, "Oh, hi. I almost didn't recognize you. I think you're a little heavier than the last time I saw you."

You know the Bible verse that says, "**Before a word is on my tongue, you know it completely, O Lord**" (Psalm 139:4 NIV)? Too bad I hadn't prayed that verse—but I'm thankful God kept me out of trouble anyway.

Both of these passing comments were made many years ago. Obviously, I've never forgotten them. It resembles what my son said the day I forgot to help in his kindergarten classroom. When I asked his forgiveness, he replied, "It's on cement in my brain." That's sort of funny from a five-year-old. Not so much from a fifty-year-old.

We hold on to some of the craziest memories, don't we? We remember frivolous things people said or did. Maybe we need a pity party every now and then. Possibly Satan is lingering at our thresholds, whispering about things from our pasts.

While some issues are trivial, like weight gain, some memories can be quite painful. So painful they make a logical excuse for a pity party. In previous days, we've mentioned how others can hurt us, emotionally beat us up, and leave us wounded wrecks. We also know our own bad choices bring heartache and, sometimes, years of guilt. But God never intended for us to live in those memories, offenses, and remorse. It is detrimental to our emotional and physical health, plus it's just so-o-o difficult to be a beautiful woman for God with bitterness, guilt, or anger in our hearts.

It surely wouldn't have benefitted Esther to hold on to her history. Her life was difficult from the beginning. She lived as an exile in a foreign land, experienced her parents' deaths, moved to a foreign palace, and took on the burden caused by Haman's evil actions. All this could very well have been cemented onto her brain.

Scripture doesn't say so directly, but I wonder whether, instead of living in bitterness and anger, she let God be God in her life. She accepted her position at the palace and then allowed God to deal with Haman. She did her part by being willing to be used and then trusted God with the results. Thank you, Esther, for our lesson on leaving the ugly behind and for giving us the first encouragement on diving into our new lives of beautiful obedience.

So how do we forget the past, accept the present, and let go of the hurt? Consider this from Psalm 103:1–5, 17–18:

> Praise the Lord, O my soul; all my inmost being, praise his holy name. Praise the Lord, O my soul, and forget not all his benefits—who forgives all your sins and heals all your diseases, who redeems your life from the pit and crowns you with love and compassion, who satisfies your desires with good things so that your youth is renewed like the eagle's. . . . But from everlasting to everlasting the Lord's love is with those who fear him, and his righteousness with their children's children—with those who keep his covenant and remember to obey his precepts (NIV).

Start with praise. You may be thinking, *Oh, sure. Praise God after what has happened to me?* Before you think this is impossible, let's consider King David who wrote these praises. He was no stranger to pit dwelling. He faced jealous brothers, fought a nine-foot giant, ran for his life from King Saul, committed murder, endured the death of a son, and lived with strained relationships between his children. Yet he continued to seek God in spite of the bad choices he made and others' evil toward him. He simply chose to praise God.

Remember the benefits. We forget the wrong things sometimes. We should be forgetting the trivial stuff that doesn't really matter. And if we did, all the negatives we hold tightly would be eliminated. But what about our genuine hurts and sorrows? This psalm tells us to **"forget not all his benefits."** Put in the positive, we are to remember God's benefits. This psalm lists some benefits: God forgives, God heals, God redeems, God energizes, and God sustains those who obey him. God is truly sufficient. If we seize and surrender those hurtful, negative experiences to God and embrace his benefits, praise just might roll off our tongues.

Forgive where necessary. This psalm reminds us that God's love and power for living are for those who obey His precepts (his principles and instructions for living). One of God's precepts is to forgive others. I often have to remind myself that forgiveness does not endorse the behavior. If it did, there would be no need for me to forgive. Forgiveness acknowledges a wrong committed and moves me forward. It takes a weight off my heart. God wants to shower us with grace and love, but we have the responsibility to live in obedience to all his laws.

Forge ahead. Have you seen an eagle fly? It seems so effortless, so peaceful, yet so powerful. This is the picture we are given of how God renews our strength to forge ahead in life. We can move ahead in peace and power as we leave the ugly behind. But it starts with a choice by us. God has already done his part. He's offered his love, forgiveness, healing, and strength. We then have to choose to embrace it.

Forgetting, forgiving, and forging is the first step in our makeover plan. Esther would be excited for us to follow her example to move on in spite of what life throws our way. Let's see what else is next.

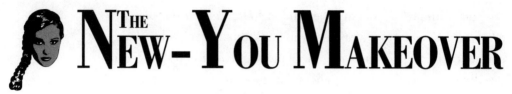

THE NEW-YOU MAKEOVER

How often do I praise God without asking for anything?

Do I believe God is sufficient for forgiveness, healing, and restoration?

Whom do I need to forgive?

What do I need to leave behind in order to move forward?

_____

_____

_____

_____

_____

_____

_____

_____

_____

_____

_____

_____

TIMELESS BEAUTY
SOURCE

ETERNAL POWER

I have to be honest: sometimes it's hard for me to move ahead. For Pete's
sake, I've held onto some of those grudges and nursed those hurts for
a long time now. And to move on might mean that I would have to . . .
change!

Change can be scary. For instance, in my little beauty world, one
of the hardest things for me to change is my hairstylist. When you're as
compulsively hair obsessed as I am, a change of stylist ranks as scary as
bungee jumping from the Golden Gate Bridge. After finding someone who
understands my hair better than me and who puts up with my HOCD, I'm
ready to take the vow " 'Til death do us part." She not only understands
my hair, she also humors me. I sit in her chair, contemplate a new style,
and then say, "My hair needs to say something."

She always responds, "And what would you like your hair to say this
time?"

Then there are purse changes. Fashion-conscious women use purses
as statements, much like I do with my hair. This confuses me. I know
what I want my hair to say. It has to say casual and, fun, yet classy. (Stop
laughing.) But I'm not sure what I'd want my purse to say about me.
Anything nice—or classy—it might say would be thoroughly undermined
when you peeked inside and saw the chaos. My husband shudders when
I say, "Go ahead and look for it—it's in my purse." He's not a real trooper
for this kind of uncharted territory.

There's another thing about purses. Many women change their purses
to match their outfits. Most days it's a chore just to locate my purse before
I leave the house, much less have the time to change the contents. And
changing purses would mean I would actually have to own more than one

purse. My philosophy: one purse, basic color, get out of the house in a hurry. (Now, if you're talking about changing shoes, that's a different story for another day!)

Change can be hard. Even when we know we need to change, even when it would be beneficial and help us follow God more closely, sometimes change seems impossible or, at the very least, overwhelming.

But even though making changes can be difficult for us, one thing hasn't and will never change: God is forever the same. Perhaps the most comforting truth I've gleaned from the book of Esther is that her God is the same God I serve today. The God of 460 BC is the God of the twenty-first century. God doesn't change—and, in this case, unchanging is good news!

If Esther were here, I think she might say something like, "God is real. Just as he moved powerfully through Abraham, Isaac, and Jacob, he worked through me, and he can work through you. If he can use a mere orphan like me, he can help you fulfill his plan for your life. Just trust and be willing to step out in faith, no matter how hard it is."

The paradox is that God's unchanging nature is what helps us change. It's what we can count on when we need courage to forgive, the determination to leave the past behind, or simply the strength to keep following God in beautiful obedience.

Take confidence from these Scriptures:

"**God is not a man, that he should lie, nor a son of man, that he should change his mind. Does he speak and then not act? Does he promise and not fulfill?**" (Numbers 23:19 NIV).

"**I the Lord do not change**" (Malachi 3:6 NIV).

"**Jesus Christ is the same yesterday and today and forever**" (Hebrews 13:8 NIV).

God's nature and promises are consistent and reliable. If he promised to always be with us, he is. If he promised to give us the strength to do all he asks, he will. And if he declared he is the same from eternity past to eternity future, embrace it.

One scary thing about change is that it involves the unknown. Questions arise like, What if I extend forgiveness and the other person is still hateful to me? What if I forgive myself and I mess up again? What if I dig deep in my heart to forget about my past and get dragged through the pain again? What if I decide to start living in radical, beautiful obedience to God and others don't understand or accept my new lifestyle?

We don't always know what's around the corner when we take a step of faith, but God does. So who greater to partner with than the one who knows everything? God knows whether you'll face ridicule, rejection, or have a hard time putting one foot in front of the other. That's why he promised a long time ago to be our unchanging, timeless source of beauty.

It's amazing what we put our trust in today. We believe a cream prevents wrinkles and makes us look younger. We trust the right outfit to give us confidence for the job interview. We even believe that the name on our purses, shoes, or dresses helps our image. But we don't trust the maker of the entire universe to help us change our attitudes or behavior?

Let's get this in perspective. God is who helps us accomplish things for eternity. Our youthful skin will eventually fade. Jobs will end. And unless we're the Israelites traveling through the wilderness, our shoes are going to wear out no matter whose name is on them. But the things we do for the kingdom of God will last forever.

Maybe I should mention something else that never changes: no one else can make changes for us. Our stylist can give us a new 'do, and our fashion-savvy friends can help us with a wardrobe makeover. But issues of the heart are God's territory. In fact, they are his specialty. He created us and knows us inside and out. Further, he's the one who knows exactly the changes we need to follow him more closely.

Now is a great time for change.

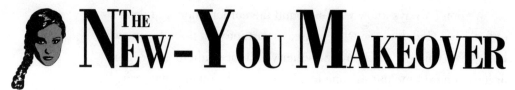

THE NEW-YOU MAKEOVER

What scares me most about change?

What have I been holding on to for way too long?

Do I need to change friends? The way I think? The way I talk? Any activities?

Am I living so I can give a responsible account of my life to my Savior?

_____

_____

_____

_____

_____

_____

_____

_____

_____

_____

_____

_____

_____

BEAUTY AND THE BEST

THRIVE, DON'T JUST SURVIVE

"OK, let's get the dastardly deed done," I said as I plopped into my hairapist's chair. At times like this, I was glad she owned her own shop and we could have some privacy.

She put on her stylist coat and reclined the chair. I laid back and braced myself with feet propped up on the counter in front of me. She must have sensed my apprehension. After all, she is my hairapist. And we'd been through this many times—too many times for my liking.

"Karen, why don't you let me wax your eyebrows. It would be a lot easier."

"What? And rip that hot wax off my skin? No way." I folded my arms across my chest.

"OK then. I'll pull them out—one by one," she replied. Did I sense villainy in her voice today?

She grabbed her tweezers. I closed my eyes, held my breath, and waited for the first pluck. Plink. I squirmed and moaned. But she just kept plucking.

She knows our routine: She plucks, I moan. She begins diversion conversation, I answer between squirms. And what seems like hours later, she raises the chair and I look in the mirror.

"How's that?" she asks as I examine my newly groomed eyebrows.

"Beautiful. We should do this more often," I answer with a smirk.

I'm not sure why God gave me such bushy eyebrows. I'm sure there's a lesson somewhere. And if I figure it out, I'll let you know. All I know is that, for now, plucking eyebrows is a necessary evil. But oh, what I'll do for beauty's sake.

Sometimes I think I approach following God's plan and this whole obedience issue in the same manner. I do love God. But sometimes I'm not careful, and my quest to follow God becomes more like a burden. I'll do it to be obedient, but I brace myself because I assume somewhere along the way God's plan is going to hurt.

Do you ever feel that way? You know you'll obey God, but it becomes more of a duty, a requirement, or just what's expected of you. If so, you're like me, and you realize the joy of obedience is gone. Following God has been reduced to a mere business transaction.

When that happens, I refocus on the words of Jesus, **"The thief comes only to steal and kill and destroy; I have come that they may have life, and have it to the full"** (John 10:10 NIV). I don't believe for a New York beauty minute that Jesus died so I would be miserable following him. Instead, Jesus took my misery on the cross so that I could have an abundant life, filled with all that God has to offer.

Oh, I can be an expert at getting all that's offered, especially with my beauty products. I strategically prop all my bottles upside down so I can coax out every last bit of beauty power I paid for. Every drop of cream and lotion is vital because, somewhere, a wrinkle needs straightening and some cellulite is forming. I thump shampoo bottles on the tub just knowing more goodness is hiding along the sides. Don't tell anyone, but I've even been known to cut the bottles in half to get out all I can.

Maybe you're thinking, *That's fine for beauty products, but how do I get all I can out of this life, experience joy, and live abundantly as a new woman in beautiful obedience?*

So glad you brought that up. Let's think about a few things:

We can learn through everything. There will be problems on the journey, but the problems don't define God's will for our lives. Rather, we use problems to draw closer to God or to help someone else who struggles like us. **"Praise be to the God and Father of our Lord Jesus Christ, the Father of compassion and the God of all comfort, who comforts us in all our troubles, so that we can comfort those in any trouble with the comfort we ourselves have received from God"** (2 Corinthians 1:3–4 NIV). Learn the beauty lesson and pay it forward.

Redefining obedience. Obedience gets a bad rap in our culture. It seems synonymous with subservience, being walked on, or inferiority. But let's face it, for peace and order we need authority, rules, and boundaries. Otherwise there would be chaos. We can be thankful that the authority who plans our lives as God's children is gracious, loving, and compassionate. Even the author who wrote a book of laments acknowledges, **"Because of the Lord's great love we are not consumed, for his compassions never fail. They are new every morning; great is your faithfulness"** (Lamentations 3:22–23 NIV). Obedience is a positive thing.

Speaking of boundaries. This is another misunderstood word, especially when it comes to Christian living. Some people think following God is a life of thou-shalt-nots. But a biblical view is that followers of Jesus receive the abundant life balanced with protection as they stay within God's safe boundaries. There are reasons beyond our knowledge why God told us to refrain from certain activities. Crossing God's boundaries can be just as dangerous as crossing that yellow dotted line down the middle of the highway that defines everyone's driving spaces. **"Lord, you have assigned me my portion and my cup; you have made my lot secure. The boundary lines have fallen for me in pleasant places"** (Psalm 16:5–6 NIV). Boundaries create security.

It's really about God. The abundant life is a great gift, but let's never forget this life is compliments of the creator of the universe. It all started with God, and he made us so we would glorify and honor him. He put everything in us we need, he initiated the relationship with us, and he sustains us day after day. Jesus said it best (no surprise!) as he prayed shortly before his death, **"Father, the time has come. Glorify your Son, so that your Son may glorify you. For you granted him authority over all people that he might give eternal life to all those you have given him. Now this is eternal life: that they may know you, the only true God, and Jesus Christ, whom you have sent. I have brought you glory on earth by completing the work you gave me to do"** (John 17:1–4 NIV.) Even Jesus brought glory to God.

Arrogant and evil Haman was all about getting all he could—for himself. If you'll remember, that didn't work out so well for him. Esther and Mordecai risked their lives to follow God and lived to tell about how God protected them. The principle of abundant, obedient living coupled with God's protection is a theme throughout the Bible. Tomorrow we'll see how beautifully God is reflected through it all.

THE NEW-YOU MAKEOVER

When have I obeyed out of duty or drudgery?

Have I ever associated the abundant life with obeying God?

How do I view the thou-shalt-nots outlined in God's Word?

Do I exhibit the joy of the abundant life as I follow God?

_____

_____

_____

_____

_____

_____

_____

_____

_____

_____

_____

_____

_____

BEAUTY REFLECTIONS

REFLECTING GOD

Ugh. Another article in my women's magazine about the importance of exercise. Why can't they give me more beauty tips, makeup instructions, and fashion advice so I can just cover it all up? But, alas, more guilt trips—uh, I mean, great tips—on how I can lose a dress size in a few months just by walking every day.

Have you ever noticed, though, that the women shown walking in the magazines always live by a beach? Either they're walking across beautiful white sand or waves are wafting in the background. It looks so serene, so tranquil, so private. But hey, I live in Kansas. My walking scenery is reduced to cars zooming by on the highway.

So I knew I'd be on public display when I started exercising to lose that dress size. Cars would zip by as I walked, but that wouldn't be a problem, would it? Well, it wasn't until I decided to see whether I could jog. After all, I ran track in junior high school. (But you can tell that was a long time ago because I said "junior high." If I'd attended "middle school," jogging would be much easier because I'd be way younger.)

Despite the years gone by, I was determined to jog. Good thing I didn't intend on jogging very far, because what happened was enough to discourage a soccer mom from driving a minivan. Theoretically, I was jogging, but gravity sucked my feet back to the ground. I kept clomping along as the cars passed by. After a few minutes (or maybe that was seconds), I noticed my upper body thrashing from side to side in synch with the stomping feet. Sweat poured down my face, and I thought, *What a sight I must be to these people driving by.*

My feet pounded the pavement like free-falling weights. My brow furrowed, I squinted from exhaustion, and my throat made guttural sounds. I figured I'd better stop when the moaning persisted. I couldn't imagine what the people passing by thought about this odd sight.

Why can't I look like the joggers I see when drive by? I wondered. *Those runners jog with weightless strides, defying gravity. Their feet come down gently; they run like the breeze, legs high in the air, smiling as if they're actually having fun. And they're barely dewy.* Two thoughts came to mind: gazelle and elephant. And if I couldn't be a gazelle, I'd just stick to walking.

I worry about such crazy things in my appearance. Everything from my shoes matching the season to my bushy eyebrows. But how concerned am I with what my actions look like to the world, knowing my actions reveal a lot about my relationship with God? Whether I like it or not, if I claim to follow Jesus, my behaviors can affect how others respond to him.

Sound a little radical? Check out these verses from Esther: **"In every province and in every city, wherever the edict of the king went, there was joy and gladness among the Jews, with feasting and celebrating. And many people of other nationalities became Jews because fear of the Jews had seized them. . . . And all the nobles of the provinces, the satraps, the governors and the king's administrators helped the Jews, because fear of Mordecai was prominent in the palace; his reputation spread throughout the provinces, and he became more and more powerful"** (Esther 8:17; 9:3–4 NIV84).

People observed Mordecai as he walked faithfully with his God. It was apparent he had something they didn't. His life of integrity was a witness to the power of God. Time and again in Scripture, we see how faithful obedience caused others to recognize the reality of God.

When the prophet Daniel interpreted King Nebuchadnezzar's dream, giving God the credit for the revelation, the pagan king responded, **"Surely your God is the God of gods and the Lord of kings and a revealer of mysteries, for you were able to reveal this mystery"** (Daniel 2:47 NIV).

After Shadrach, Meshach, and Abednego were thrown into a fiery furnace for their refusal to bow to an idol of gold, they emerged miraculously untouched by the fire. The same king declared, **"Praise be to the God of Shadrach, Meshach and Abednego, who has sent his** angel and rescued his servants! They trusted in him and defied the king's command and were willing to give up their lives rather than serve or worship any god except their own God" (Daniel 3:28 NIV).

Daniel was thrown into a lion's den as punishment for praying to his God. He survived unhurt also, and King Darius wrote, "I issue a decree that in every part of my kingdom people must fear and reverence the God of Daniel. For he is the living God and he endures forever" (Daniel 6:26 NIV).

One of the most powerful ways to influence others for God is to live faithfully and obediently to him, reflecting his character. If you want to help your friends and family know your God, just live a consistent, beautiful life of obedience. They will see it. They will take notice.

We have to be careful, though, that our actions aren't just for outward appearances—that we don't become consumed with what others think, as I vainly did in my jogging efforts. This became clear to me one day as I thought about beautiful obedience. I asked God, "What is the deepest meaning of 'walking in obedience'?"

God clearly answered, "It's having an obedient heart."

Wow, I thought. *That's an inside job.* I suddenly realized I've done a lot of looking good on the outside. I've tried to be a supportive wife, a godly mom, and a faithful servant at church. But God wants obedience clear down to my heart. He desires that I long to be the woman he wants—not just one going through the motions. He wants my heart as beautiful as my actions.

What does a beautiful heart look like? It's a heart full of the character of God and a willingness to put character into action. And how do I know whether I'm operating from a beautiful heart or simply from a need to look good, godly, and proper on the outside? The answer is whether I'm determined to do the right thing and not care if I'm thanked or even appreciated by the world around me.

Often, if we're obedient, especially in the smallest details, we won't receive recognition for our efforts. Don't get me wrong—people are watching, and some might make declarations like the kings who honored Daniel and his friends. But if you're counting on that, you need to have a heart checkup.

When we have our hearts fully turned toward God, it's much easier to follow his will. And when we do this, especially in the tough times, we reflect a beauty that tells the world we serve a great big God.

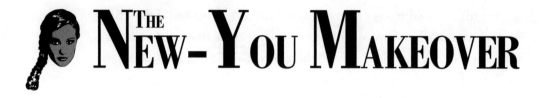

THE NEW-YOU MAKEOVER

When do I worry most about what others think?

If others were to define God by my actions, what would they say?

Can I honestly say I have a beautiful heart?

How can my life be more reflective of God's character?

_____

_____

_____

_____

_____

_____

_____

_____

_____

_____

_____

_____

_____

_____

BEAUTY SABOTAGED

NOT PERFECT YET

I anxiously took off on a personal retreat to get a project finished. The campground where I was headed would give me a quiet place to work and wide open spaces for enjoying God's beautiful world. It also would give me a great place to exercise away from zooming cars, as I was still trying to lose that dress size.

The cheerful twenty-something camp manager knew I wanted to walk and asked one afternoon, "Would you like me to show you the ridge path?"

"Sure," I said.

"Great. I'd better get my boots." She headed to her room to change.

Boots? For exercise? Maybe that should have been my first clue that this would be no beauty walk in the park. And maybe my second clue should have been the word *mountain* in the campground's name.

She returned, and we walked a little way and then headed up a slight hill. *This ain't nothing,* I thought. *I've been exercising for a few months now. I'm old enough to be her mother, but I can keep up with this youngster.*

That hill leveled out, and we started up another one. *No problem. I'm in such good shape she might even be impressed. After all, it's not like we're jogging.* This hill was a bit longer, though. I felt my heart beat harder and my breathing get heavier. *I can do this. I'm in shape,* I thought as I panted.

Just when I thought we could rest, another hill loomed in front of us. My exercise pal didn't miss a beat. She trudged in her boots, and I shuffled my tennis shoes as fast as I could to convince her, me, and God that I was in control of the situation. Then I felt a sharp pain in my lungs I hadn't experienced since my jogger-wannabe episode. If you're not getting the picture yet, I ask, does off-roading mean anything to you?

We finally got to level ground. I tried not to pant too noticeably. She asked, "So, do you want to talk about the project you're working on?"

I would if I could breathe! Somehow I found the air and composure to say, "Sure." And the rest is history. I regained my breath, the hike was beautiful, and I made a new friend. And guess what? I got up the next morning and headed for that mountain.

You know, sometimes hiking through life we think we're spiritually toned and conditioned. Maybe we are. We've been walking in beautiful obedience and are ready for anything. Then we hit some rough terrain. *That's OK,* we think. *Problems will come. I can handle this.* But the problems turn out to be bigger than we thought, and soon we run out of spiritual breath and maybe even stumble and fall.

Some of you reading right now may have just begun your own makeover. You are praying more, reading more of God's Word, and listening more to the Holy Spirit. You have your friends lined up to encourage and inspire you. Life will be good. It's the New You.

Be prepared. There will be some bad-hair days. In fact, your choice to renew your efforts and walk in beautiful obedience really ticked off Satan. You might be knocked down by temptation, say words you shouldn't, or act contrary to God's desire. The best thing is to get back up and grab on to Jesus again. Ask for forgiveness and receive God's mercy. I simply don't know any other way to continue on except through the grace God extends to us.

There will be difficult decisions as you continue to stay faithful to God. It reminds me of a decision I had to make when I climbed the mountain that next morning by myself. I took a different path and came to a fork in the road. One way went up another hill, the other was lower ground. *I'm going to take the high road,* I thought, and began my ascent. Secretly I hoped it worked those thighs a little harder.

When faced with choices on our journey of following God, it's always best when we take the high road. The world is full of people who choose the low road and compromise the journey. Sometimes it's followers of God who choose the lazy spiritual life, just barely investing in a relationship with God. I know. I've done just that. The results are spiritual anemia, apathy, and amnesia. And trust me on this one, it's anything but beautiful.

The high road is hard. It requires more energy, more time, and more dependence on God. But the trip is always worth it—and you will feel better afterward. You might even strengthen a spiritual muscle or two.

Esther had a huge mountain to climb without ever leaving the palace. I'm not sure whether she preferred royal hiking boots or tennis shoes, and I doubt she had an arrogant attitude like mine. The mountain, at first, must have seemed huge—her people were under a murder edict. How do you scale a problem like that?

By taking the high road. Can you imagine the peace she felt after it was all over? It was definitely worth any tired feet or dewy brows.

Think about these verses as you head for the high road: **"For this very reason, make every effort to add to your faith goodness; and to goodness, knowledge; and to knowledge, self-control; and to self-control, perseverance; and to perseverance, godliness; and to godliness, brotherly kindness; and to brotherly kindness, love. For it you possess these qualities in increasing measure, they will keep you from being ineffective and unproductive in your knowledge of our Lord Jesus Christ"** (2 Peter 1:5–8 NIV84).

Did you catch that word *effort*? No one ever said following God would be easy—or natural. The more we imitate godly character, the more easily obedience will come. But we won't ever get to stop trying to be like Jesus until we reach the highest mountain—heaven.

Speaking of heaven—let's party!

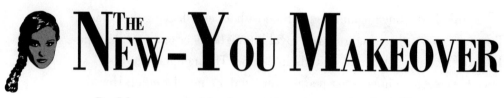

THE NEW-YOU MAKEOVER

Do I have any pride that might trip me up when I least expect?

When I've spiritually fallen before, what did I do to get back up? Did that help?

What high road do I need to take?

What trait from 2 Peter 1:5–8 should I work on right now?

_____

_____

_____

_____

_____

_____

_____

_____

_____

_____

_____

_____

LET'S PARTY!

PURIM STYLE

My six-year-old daughter played among the bubbles in the bathtub while I stood nearby. She ran the washcloth over her legs and then paused. With a heavy sigh, she scrutinized her legs and asked, "How am I going to get a boyfriend with all these bruises on my legs?"

Boyfriend? Age six? In a panic, I dismissed the bruises issue and headed straight for the boyfriend question. Wanting her to be friends with girls as well as boys, I answered, "I'll just tell you what my mom told me when I was little. There's a lot of fishies in the sea."

She looked up at me and furrowed her brow. After a long silence she asked, "Did you know what your mom meant when she said that?"

OK, so I don't excel in every teachable moment. But she did understand another story I told her quite often. As a little girl, she liked to play dress up and put on makeup. While she was decked out with lipstick and some eye shadow, I'd tell her the story of the "very, very pretty lady." It went something like this: "The very, very pretty lady drove up in her limousine. She stepped out of the car into the crowd, and everyone *oohed* and *aahed* at her beauty. She wore a beautiful red dress with sparkly shoes. Her face was perfect, with glimmering eye shadow and rosy lips. Everyone thought she was the most beautiful lady in the world. Then someone bumped her. Out of her mouth came the most horrible, unkind, ugly words ever heard. All of a sudden people saw her for who she really was, and she didn't seem so beautiful anymore."

Even as a young child, my daughter absorbed the story with amazement. And often when she played dress up, she'd say, "Tell me the story of the very, very pretty lady."

Do you ever feel like there's that little girl inside of you? There is in me. The one who worries if she looks pretty, likes to play dress up, and

185

begs mom to remind her of what pretty really is. Maybe we never outgrow the desire to feel beautiful. However, at some point we have to acquire a grown-up view of what beauty really is. And for that we look to our heavenly Father.

Imagine this: All the women of the world gathered into one huge arena at a Beauty-Is-Us Conference. God is the keynote speaker. I think he would say something like this: "Ladies, I love you more than you can fathom. I created each of you special, with distinct purposes to fulfill. I'm so sorry for what others have done to you. I will take care of that. I'm also sad over the bad choices you've made. And that's why I sent my Son to die for you. But now I want you to move on! I want you to celebrate the plans I made for you. And I want you to know that, no matter what you look like on the outside, you are beautiful when your hearts follow me. Come on and celebrate the women I made you to be."

I would never try to put words in God's mouth, so consider these verses as supporting evidence:

"This is how God showed his love among us: he sent his one and only Son into the world that we might live through him" (1 John 4:9 NIV).

"For we are God's workmanship, created in Christ Jesus to do good works" (Ephesians 2:10 NIV 84).

"Come to me [Jesus], all you who are weary and burdened, and I will give you rest" (Matthew 11:28 NIV).

"Jesus replied, 'No one who puts a hand to the plow and looks back is fit for service in the kingdom of God'" (Luke 9:62 NIV).

God knows following him in beautiful obedience isn't always easy. But he's always with us. Maybe that's why he insisted that the people in the Old Testament celebrate and commemorate events and victories along the journey. The Jews were told to host holidays and feasts, including Passover, the Feast of Trumpets, and the Day of Atonement. These festivals sometimes included times of confession, but there was plenty of celebrating too. We also remember how Joshua was instructed to place twelve stones in the Jordan River to commemorate and celebrate the Jews' victorious passage across the flooded river on their way to the Promised Land.

There was celebrating in Esther's time too. Her brave actions allowed the Jews to defend themselves against their enemies. The Jews fought back and won. Her people were saved!

After this victory, Esther and Mordecai established an annual time of celebration. They called it Purim. The party reminded the Jews of success over their enemies and how their sorrow was turned into joy and celebration. For two days each year, they were to celebrate by giving gifts and holding a feast that would put any church potluck to shame.

Maybe we should throw a few more celebrations as we follow God. We can rejoice in the plan he has charted for our lives, knowing he knows best. We can thank him that he gives us comfort and wisdom as we deal with our problems. We can celebrate his forgiveness when we veer off his path and act ugly.

However, my biggest cause to celebrate is how he loves me no matter what I weigh, how many wrinkles I have, or whether I wear lime green capris.

Purim probably also reminded the Jews that tough times don't last forever. We need to remember there will be a day when we won't have to deal with the struggles of life! When we stand before our God, possibly with Queen Esther at our side, God won't check for designer labels on our blouses or ask us to step on the scales. But Scripture indicates we will be responsible for how we lived our lives, from the way we treated others to how we used our God-given abilities and talents.

And you know what, girlfriends? Looking beautiful is great, even though some days it's really hard for me. I'm going to keep using my cellulite-removing lotion and the perfect foundation and scheduling regular visits with my hairapist. I want to go down looking as good as I can. However, can I impose my superhuman strength one more time? I want to challenge you to celebrate this: no matter what you think you look like, no matter what the scales say, and even if you don't look like the magazine models (who does?)—you are beautiful to God when you walk beside him in beautiful obedience.

You are more than just a pretty face!

MY CELEBRATIONS: Record thoughts or milestones to celebrate what you have experienced on your beauty journey.

DAY
31

MY CELEBRATIONS

NOTES

1. "Oops! Australia's Next Top Model Crowns Wrong Winner," http://www.usmagazine.com/stylebeauty/news/oops-australias-next-top-model-crowns-wrong-winner-2010299.

2. "Pursuit of Youth Isn't Always Pretty," Julia Sommerfeld, http://www.msnbc.msn.com/id/23359042/ns/health-aging/.

3. "Look Younger by Monday," Ginger Otis, http://www.goodhousekeeping.com/beauty/skin/younger-by-monday?click=main_sr.

4. Matthew Henry, A Commentary on the Whole Bible, Vol. 2 (Iowa City, IA: World Bible Publishers, 1980), 1121.

5. "Why You Should Fast," Bill Bright http://www.ccci.org/training-and-growth/devotional-life/personal-guide-to-fasting/02-why-you-should-fast.htm.

6. "What Scares Men about Women," Laura Hagans Smith, http://lifestyle.msn.com/relationships/articlematch.aspx?cp-document id=25781580&GT1=32023.

APPLYING THE FOUNDATION

If you want to start a new beautiful life of obedience with a foundation built on Jesus Christ, it can be as simple as A-B-C-D:

A. Admit you have sinned and ask for forgiveness. "**For all have sinned and fall short of the glory of God**" (Romans 3:23 NIV).

B. Believe Jesus died on the cross to pay the penalty for your sin. "**For God so loved the world that he gave his one and only Son, that whoever believes in him shall not perish but have eternal life**" (John 3:16 NIV).

C. Confess Jesus as Savior and Lord of your life. "**If you confess with your mouth, 'Jesus is Lord,' and believe in your heart that God raised him from the dead, you will be saved**" (Romans 10:9 NIV).

D. Decide to live for Jesus. "**To this you were called, because Christ suffered for you, leaving you an example, that you should follow in his steps**" (1 Peter 2:21 NIV).

You can pray and tell God something like this: "God, I am sorry for my sin. I believe you sent your Son, Jesus, to die on the cross so I could be forgiven and live with you forever. I confess that Jesus is my Savior, and I invite him to be my Lord, the new Master of my life. Thank you for saving me, and help me to live for you."

If you say this prayer, tell other Christians so they can encourage you. Find a church that teaches the Bible and serve with the abilities God has given you.

You will never regret making the most beautiful decision of your life.